purpose in paralysis

from chronic pain to universal gain

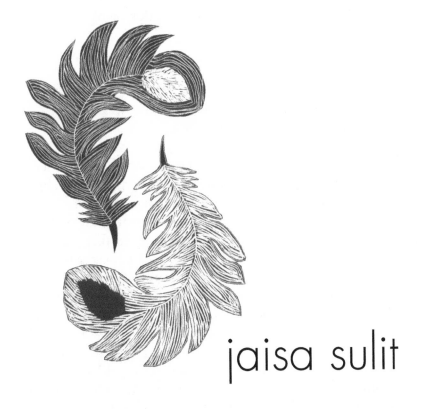

jaisa sulit

Published by Jaisa Sulit, May, 2018
ISBN: 9780995984202

Editor: Nina Shoroplova
Typeset: Greg Salisbury
Book Cover Design: Judith Mazari and Erin Taniguchi
Portrait Photographer: Devon Slack

For everyone who played a role in my healing after the accident, especially my mother and my father.

Contents

Part V: An Overachiever Accepts What Can't Be Achieved

Foreword

When Jaisa Sulit first asked me to write the foreword to her book, my response was "No, I'm the wrong person. I'm your editor. You want someone else to write your foreword." But then I started to recognize how well I understood her journey. Apart from the specifics of what launched us on our wellness and spiritual journeys, both Jaisa and I began as therapists working within the field of Western medicine, I as a physiotherapist, she as an occupational therapist. From our medical education, we both looked askance at Eastern modalities with their focus on the energy body, the soul, the spirit, past lives, and even reincarnation.

And so I agreed to try to capture the elements of Jaisa Sulit's book in a foreword. After all, she had me at "It's all about relationships."

What happens when an occupational therapist working in the field of neurological rehabilitation undergoes a spinal cord injury herself, one that requires her to work with physiotherapists, occupational therapists, chiropractors, massage therapists, body workers, a dietician, a physiatrist (a doctor who specializes in rehabilitation), a social worker, a case manager, and two caring lawyers?

Jaisa doesn't experience the journey that we would expect. Her journey is not merely about learning to walk the walk (with a walker, then canes, hiking sticks, and ankle foot braces); it's about dealing with pain management, depression, and a drive to overachieve and be perfect—and learning how judgmental her Newtonian education had made her.

It's also far more than that.

More importantly, Jaisa's journey became—and still continues to become—an opportunity to heal her physical being, her emotional inner child, her unclaimed soul, her spirit that has lived lives both good and bad. It's an opportunity to acknowledge the lives of her Filipino ancestors, especially the ancient healers whose stories were lost through colonization.

In the ongoing process of healing herself, Jaisa has become a profound healer for others, using the wisdom of the mindfulness-based stress reduction program she learned and now teaches.

She also talks the talk. Writing in its many forms—journaling as a girl, writing poetry, blogging, and now authoring—are healing practices that she is bringing into the public arena as a spoken word artist, an improv and comedy student, and a keynote speaker in Canada and Mexico.

As a child, Jaisa took jazz, tap, lyrical ballet, and Hawaiian dance classes. Pre-injury, she became a barefoot Filipina folk dancer, loving the precision and challenge of being a *tinikling* dancer, jumping between bamboo sticks that close together on every beat of the music. Now, post-injury and knowing how her recovery has taken her beyond the limitations of her previous life, she holds open the door of possibility in which barefoot dancing will once again be among the activities she can enjoy.

For a few years, Jaisa lived in my neighbourhood—the West End of Vancouver. She loved walking on the sand, cycling the Stanley Park trails, climbing the North Shore mountains. Now back in Toronto, Jaisa is ready to embrace life with all its challenges and darkness, because she knows how to connect with the Universe, with Source, with Father Sky and Mother Earth, and with "that thing" that unites us through our breath and makes life fall into place.

Nina Shoroplova, physiotherapist (retired), book editor, and author of *Cattle Ranch*, *Trust the Mystery*, and *Spiraling Self-Awareness*, March 2018

Author's Preface

*Strong like a river that knows its course, the river that flows
from source.*
Murray Kyle

I initially wanted to write a book that would help others to
heal. But as life would have it, the narrative process forced me
to see that I had wounds yet to tend to. I needed to heal myself
first.

So alas, this is not a how-to book. It's a how-I've-done-it
book.

How I've learned to reinhabit this human body.

How I've come to live well with pain.

How I've reclaimed parts of myself I once judged and
exiled.

And how I've reconnected with my higher authentic self
and the truth of who I really am.

We are all mirrors to each other's lives. So just as I see myself
in others, my hope in sharing my experiences so vulnerably
with you is that you may see yourself in me and, just as I have,
meet parts of yourself still waiting to be held.

Part I

Broken and In Pain

1

Getting What I Asked For

I Put On a Fake Smile

Disconnected from myself, it took one year for me to finally acknowledge my grief and cry.

I was out for brunch with two girlfriends—both of them marathon runners—and they were talking about their upcoming races and how their trainings were going. I too had been a runner; I was at the peak of my training when I sustained a spinal cord injury. So it was hard for me to hear my friends speak of all the things I wasn't able to do, for at that point in time I needed two canes to walk and a wheelchair for travelling long distances.

As I listened to my friends share their experiences of being part of their running clubs, I put on a fake smile. I was sad. I felt left out and I was jealous because I wanted to be a part of their running community as well. But I felt bad for feeling how I felt, so I tried hard to keep smiling. But repressing those emotions was the last straw, because hard as I tried to hide them, tears started to well up in my eyes.

"I don't want them to feel bad for me. I should be positive," I thought to myself. I didn't want them to know I was sad and I definitely did not want to rain on their parade. But regardless of my thoughts and my effort to smile, the river of tears had already begun to flow and there was no stopping it.

Despite sitting in a full restaurant with people all around us, I cried aloud.

I Needed Change

Just two years before that emotional breakdown, I found myself in a state of confusion and desperation. With a habit of living inside my head instead of in my body, I had no sense of my true authentic self. Unable to embody life, I was unfulfilled by every career and every romantic partner that I chose. By age thirty I was contemplating a third career change and had already travelled to thirty countries. Looking outwards for acceptance, I was unhappy with who I was; but no one could ever tell.
I was good at smiling.
On August 25, 2010, I pulled out my journal and I wrote a letter asking the universe to change me.

> *August 25, 2010*
> *Dear God,*
> *Please help me to stop judging so much. I want to live with more love. I ask you to bless me, my parents, friends and foes with your guidance.*

On August 28, 2010, just three days after I journaled that request, I received the change that I had asked for. While it was not the kind of change I expected, it was exactly the change that I needed.

It was a sunny Saturday afternoon and I was at a motorcycle school, learning to ride a GZ250 Suzuki Marauder. While I had grown up from a toddler riding with my dad on his motorcycles as a passenger, this was my first time learning how to ride a motorcycle myself. I found the bike too heavy for my ninety-nine-pound body, so by the end of the day I was feeling tired and my hands were sore from holding onto the large hand grips and throttle.

The instructor gave my class some free time to go over the various motorcycle skills we had learned that day. Though my body was tired, my mind was committed to perfecting my ability to make left and right turns. With only a few minutes left before the end of class, I decided to do one more round of left turns inside the school's parking lot.

I recall the narrative in my mind: "Okay, turn left. Good. Now change gears. Drive straight. Another left turn coming up. Prepare. Change gears. Let's do this. Turn left."

As I attempted to make that left turn, for some reason, perhaps fatigue, my left hand let go of the throttle.

Fear came instantly. Instead of completing the left turn, I was now heading straight toward a curb and a chain-link fence.

"I don't know what to do!" Accelerating too fast, I had no time to think of how to regain control of the bike, so I did the only thing I could do.

I closed my eyes and surrendered.

"I allow," I thought to myself. Time then slowed down as I watched my eyelids lower to a close. In the following brief yet prolonged moments, I sensed some peace.

Boom! My bike hit the curb.

"I'm in the air," I thought as my body flipped upside down and flew ten feet across the air.

Boom! My body hit the chain-link fence.

Final boom! I landed on the ground. As I opened my eyes, I was surprised.

"I'm alive!" I was lying on my left side in a fetal position and conscious of what was going on around me.

Wheeeeee! A whistle was blown by the course instructors to indicate all student riders were to stop.

"I can't move my legs," I thought to myself. It appeared I was paralyzed from the waist down, but I must have been in shock, because I felt no pain and no sense of stress. Oddly, I was feeling drawn to the vividness of the green grass I was lying on and the blue sky that I was looking up at.

"It's actually a beautiful day," I thought.

"Anak!" My dad, who was observing the class from the sidelines, ran over to me (*anak* means "daughter, son, or child" in Tagalog).

"Dad, I can't move my legs." I could sense fear in him as he heard me say those words. I was his only child and there I was, paralyzed. I then sensed him place a hand on my lower leg.

"I can feel," I thought with excitement. The ability to sense my dad's hand on my leg gave me hope, for I knew it meant that my spinal cord was not completely severed.

One of the course instructors immediately came over to me.

"I can't move my legs," I told him.

He called for an ambulance and, fortunately for me, within what felt like only five to ten minutes paramedics arrived and began attending to me. They carefully took off my helmet and replaced it with a collar around my neck.

"Oh my God," I thought as pain started to kick in in my back when the paramedics stretched my body from fetal position to lying flat on the stretcher. This pain continued to intensify during the ambulance ride. Any bump on the road brought with it sensations of knives cutting through my back.

"Go slowly! Please," I begged the paramedics.

With my body strapped securely onto the stretcher and a neck collar stabilizing my neck, all I could look at was the ceiling of the ambulance.

"That's an interesting pattern," I thought to myself as I noticed the grooved patterns on the shiny metal surface of the ceiling. Never having been in an ambulance before, I somehow found a moment of intrigue.

As I stared at the shiny grooved patterns, something happened all of a sudden. I was overcome with a feeling of peace as an insight arose from within my body.

"It's all about relationships" were the words that came to me.

"It's all about relationships?" For a brief moment I was confused. Those words had never come from me before and now here they were; a truth bomb was blowing apart my perception of the world.

"Yes! It is all about relationships!" I became overwhelmed with gratitude as clarity arose. "Even if I'm in a wheelchair for the rest of my life, I still have the most important thing in life: the ability to be in relationship—with God, with others, and with myself!" In those brief moments of realization, I did not feel any pain.

But those moments were brief. The sensation of knives cutting through my back returned as the ambulance drove over a speed bump. We were starting to slow down.

"We have arrived. That was fast," I thought. We had been driving for twenty minutes.

"Where are we?" I asked.

"We've taken you to Sunnybrook," the paramedic replied. Luckily for me, Sunnybrook Health Sciences Centre is one of the best hospitals in Canada.

She Will Never Walk Again

I was soon admitted and taken to a room where several nurses used scissors to cut off all the clothes I was wearing.

"Oh!" I thought with surprise as I felt and heard the sound of my denim jacket being cut apart. "So this is how they take patients' clothes off. That's practical," I thought with curious interest, as if I were a medical student on her first fieldwork placement. I had been working as an occupational therapist for five years, but this was my first time in Emergency; now I got to experience it as a patient.

I also got to experience pain like I never had in my life. I was scared.

Prior to surgery I had to get my back scanned for imaging, so I had to be transported some distance via the stretcher. Though I'm sure the floors were smooth, with my back being incredibly sensitive to any movement, I desperately asked the person pushing the stretcher, "Please go slowly! It really hurts."

Though I don't recall his name, I can't forget the compassionate presence of this one man who was responsible for transporting me from point A to B to C. I don't recall the words we exchanged, but I remember the way he made me feel. I felt like he genuinely cared. The way he calmly listened and responded, the way he leaned over the stretcher so that I could see his smiling face when we spoke, the way he simply paid attention to me—all made what could have been a traumatic experience somehow bearable.

After the imaging scans were complete, I was brought into a room to be prepped for surgery.

"Just take some deep breaths now," I heard. It didn't take long before the anesthesia kicked in.

For the next nine hours, orthopaedic surgeon Michael H. Ford, MD, and his team worked to save what they could of my spinal cord.

By landing on my head, I had caused a vertical compression of my spinal column. My twelfth thoracic vertebra took the force of the impact and burst into pieces, causing compression of my spinal cord by 60 percent. Dr. Ford and his team decompressed my spinal cord by removing the majority of the shattered vertebra that was causing the compression and resulting paralysis. A bone graft was then taken from my left hip to replace the twelfth thoracic vertebra. In order to support the new bone graft, two titanium rods and eight screws were permanently placed along my spine, spanning five vertebrae from the bottom of my rib cage to my pelvis.

In the hours following that surgery, I fell in and out of a heavily sedated sleep. Every time I opened my eyes, either a nurse or a doctor would be asking me how I was doing, or the face of a new family member or friend would be smiling down at me. Little did I know that the waiting room was filled with over a dozen of my friends and family and that after the surgery Dr. Ford had gone into that waiting room and told everyone that I would never walk again.

Odd as this sounds, I got the change I had asked for. What better way for a mindless neuro-rehab occupational therapist to slow down, get out of her head, and reconnect with herself … than paralysis?

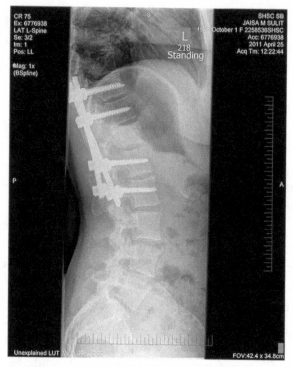

A follow up X-ray (taken six months after the accident) showing the permanent location of the two rods and eight screws in my back.

2

Pain Is a Platform

Waking Up

"Can you bend your knees?" asked someone in hospital scrubs when I finally awoke from surgery. There were several people in scrubs standing at my bedside with a look of anticipation on their faces.

I attempted to slide my left foot along the bed toward my hips, bending my left knee. Though it was slow moving, it moved. But its movement came with the sensation of knives cutting through the muscles of my back and leg. I soon learned that what I was experiencing was called neuropathic pain, which is the type of pain associated with a damaged nervous system.

"It hurts," I said. Despite the excruciating pain, I felt hope and happiness. "I can move my legs," I thought to myself. I then attempted to bend my right knee. Though its movement was also painful, I was relieved by my ability to move.

However, bending my knees was the only thing I had control of. I had minimal activation of my core trunk muscles, my leg extensors such as the buttocks and quad muscles, and little movement in my ankles and feet. Consequently, I needed two people just to help me roll from side to side in bed. I had also lost control of my bowels and bladder, so I had to rely on the use of catheters and diapers. Between my body's lack of function and the excessive neuropathic pain, the next few days were filled with horrible moments.

Fortunately, one of my best friends, Lynn Castro, knew my needs well and gifted me with a journal so that I could write my way through the tough times. My first entry was in the early morning of August 30, 2010, just two days after the accident.

> *I am still strong. I am happy. My faith in the divine is what keeps me strong. I have faith that I am loved and that I won't be put through anything that I cannot handle. Whether I am using a walker or a wheelchair, whether my pain feels like a "one out of ten" or a "ten out of ten," I know I can handle anything that comes my way. And I know that I am loved because of all the family and friends who are in my life. Through this, I am shown that I am loved.*

I then went on to make a list of everyone and everything I was thankful for, and filled four pages that morning. I went on like this each day, writing about my experiences, both the good and the bad, but always ending with a long list of what I was thankful for. Gratitude soon ended up paving the way for me to learn that from the horrible moments come the greatest opportunities.

The Growth of Something Good

The notion that pain can be a platform for the growth of something good was instilled in me by my friend Anna To, who, just a few months before my accident, gave me a piece of paper with the following passage from Romans 5:3–4 written on it: "Suffering produces perseverance; perseverance, character; and character, hope."

For some reason I kept that piece of paper in my wallet all summer, unaware that it was preparing me for the challenge that was soon to come. But just as our mistakes are our biggest teachers, my first learning experience on coping with the challenge of pain came from the failure to do so.

A week and a half into my stay at Sunnybrook Hospital, I experienced the most intense pain I have ever felt to this day. More painful than breaking my back is the pain of having a full bladder that I cannot empty on my own. One night when my bladder was starting to feel full, I pressed the button on my call bell, hoping a nurse would come to catheterize me. For what seemed like half an hour, every time I pressed the button, my call bell was turned off.

"Are they purposely ignoring me?" I worried. The pain in my bladder was sharp and burning, like hundreds of hot needles poking from the inside. "Why are they ignoring me?" I thought anxiously.

Eventually a nurse did come with an apology that they were understaffed, but it was too late. I was already traumatized. For the next week I developed fear around my call bell not being answered.

One evening later that week my mother was at my bedside when one of my godmothers came for a visit. After conversing with us for about an hour, my godmother asked my mom if she wanted to go to the cafeteria with her for a coffee. My mom turned to me and asked if she could take a break. I quickly said, "No."

I did not want to be left alone and risk feeling the pain of a full bladder that I could not empty again. With my mom beside me, I felt comfort that there would always be someone to physically retrieve a nurse for me when I needed one.

After my mom left that night, I felt the need to pull out my journal and reflect. I was feeling guilty.

I have been so concerned about pain and peeing that I've become an annoying demanding patient. "Mom, hurry! Mom, massage me! My feet hurt! I have to pee! It hurts!" My fear of pain blinded me from seeing my mom's own needs so that I didn't even allow her to have a coffee break. She didn't even get to eat a proper dinner tonight, all because I was afraid of pain.

As I wrote those words, the situation became clear to me. I had allowed pain to become a platform for the growth of my fear. And as that fear of pain grew, my potential to harm those I loved grew with it. Vowing to never let how I treated my mom that night happen again, I wrote a contract with myself promising to make pain a platform for the growth of something good.

September 4, 2010
From tonight's weakness and mistake, I grow in strength and wisdom. I promise I will never let the fear of pain bring out the worst in me again. I am not powerless in the face of fear. I am powerful because I have the power to choose to face pain and endure it with courage. I pray that I'll continue to have the strength to endure anything that happens, but I need to do my part. I will drink enough water, learn to massage myself, get enough rest, and take the pain medications when I need them.

After signing that contract with myself, I looked up from my journal and, as if pain were standing right in front of me, I looked straight at it and said in my head, "Bring it on, pain. You have got nothing on me. There is no pain so great that I will ever fear you again. So go ahead. Bring it on."

A Living Funeral

As news of my accident spread through my community, dozens of visitors came daily. The experience of seeing all these people who would change their schedules at the drop of a hat to visit me during my time of need was equivalent to the experience of a living funeral. Anyone who would have shown me love at my funeral (had I had one) I got to see in person without having to die. This was a gift because, little did everyone in my life know, there were a handful of times when I had thought about killing myself.

In the year leading to the motorcycle accident, I occasionally found myself driving in the left lane of Highway 401 thinking to myself, "It would be so easy for me to swerve my car off the highway." I fantasized about my funeral being filled with many people who would gather to mourn my passing. "Everyone will see how loved I was." Sadly, I didn't know how loved I was, for I didn't even love myself.

My chronic self-judgment had created a filter so thick that it blocked me from experiencing the reality of the love I already had in my life. But the accident gave me the funeral experience I fantasized about, and it woke me up to what I had all along—relationships. Each person that gave me love while I was in the hospital brought meaning and purpose to what I knew would be a painful road ahead. But most especially, I became aware of the depth of my parents' love. They made the biggest sacrifices in time to support me every day, helping me with my mobility, providing massages to ease my pain, and helping me with my bladder and bowel movements.

September 4, 2010

The epitome of my parents' love and support for me during these times happened today when I was in the hallway bathroom trying to have a bowel movement. The commode I was sitting on ended up being broken, so my dad had to come in to hold the commode seat down and my mom had to embrace my body to prevent me from sliding off the seat. In the midst of my bowel movement while sitting on the commode in between my mom and my dad, I thought to myself, "This is a loving family. Thank you, God."

On September 7, my *tita* Wendy Arena (tita means "aunt" in Tagalog) gave me a prayer for healing that came from the Philippines; she had printed it out especially for me. Here is a portion of that prayer.

Prayer for Healing

Lord, look upon me with eyes of mercy. May your healing Spirit rest upon me. It is through your power that I was created. Since you created me from nothing, you can certainly recreate me. Fill me with the healing power of your spirit. May your life-giving power flow into every cell of my body and into the depths of my soul. Mend what is broken. Cast out anything that should not be within me. Rebuild my brokenness. Restore my strength for service. Touch my soul with your compassion for others. Touch my heart with your courage and infinite love for all.

Though I was no longer a practising Catholic at the time there was truth resonating within me so I taped that prayer to the inside front flap of my journal and flipped to the next clean page in my journal, where I wrote another contract with myself.

How blessed am I? I cannot even attempt to describe how blessed, for any description would be limiting. I have a lot of issues but I know it's a process. As well as the fear and pain I've also felt a joy, happiness, and love like never before. I know my purpose—it is to love better. It is not enough for me to recover just so that I can go back to how I was before the accident. I need to grow physically, emotionally, and spiritually so that I can be of better service to my community.

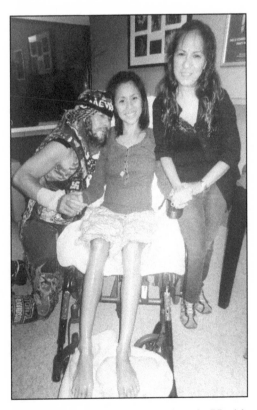

With my parents at Sunnybrook Health Sciences Centre one week after the accident.

3

Not Recovering as I Planned

Limitation and Irritation

"You're going to run again," said Mayleen, one of my best friends.

I believed it. In fact, I also believed that in just one year after the accident I would be back at work full time. Over five years of working in several neuro-rehab settings with patients exhibiting paralysis had taught me that neuroplasticity is for real.

"Neuro" refers to our neurons (nerve cells) and "plastic" refers to the quality of being changeable. So "neuroplasticity" points to the ability of the neurons in our nervous system to rewire and reorganize themselves based on the experiences we practise. What we train we neurally ingrain. What we practise we become. Put simply, neuroplasticity allows us to learn to do things we didn't think we could do. So just as I had helped my patients practise rewiring their bodies, I practised relearning how to get out of bed, stand, crawl, walk, climb stairs, and even empty my bladder again.

After two weeks at Sunnybrook, I was transferred to the Toronto Rehabilitation Institute (TRI) at Lyndhurst Centre (now part of the University Health Network), where I completed three months of therapy as an inpatient. Afterwards

I was discharged home and continued my rehabilitation as an outpatient at TRI two to three days a week, while the other two to three days I supplemented with additional therapy through my insurance funding. I had a great team, comprising physiotherapists, occupational therapists, therapy assistants, chiropractors, massage therapists, a dietician, a physiatrist (a doctor who specializes in rehabilitation), a social worker, a case manager, and two caring lawyers who managed my insurance claim.

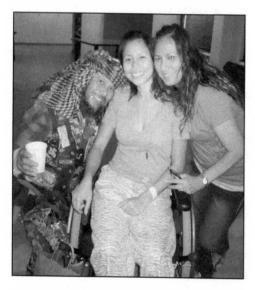

My parents supported me daily while I was an inpatient at the Toronto Rehabilitation Institute.

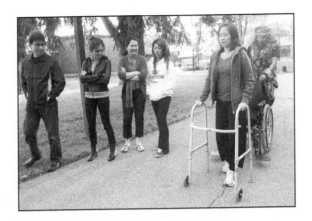

Learning to walk with a two-wheeled walker with the support of my father who is pushing the wheelchair. Uncle Ogie, Aunty Cor, and my cousins Stephanie and Sarah are alongside.

With the help of this multidisciplinary team, within the first year after the accident I had progressed from the use of a wheelchair to a walker, to two canes, to the use of just two hiking sticks. Some would think I was recovering well, but it was really a matter of perspective, because in my eyes I was nowhere close to my goal of running and returning to work.

Instead, I was starting to feel depressed.

My new reality of life with a disability was hard to accept. For instance, I couldn't accept how I needed to wear foot braces and orthotic shoes, and use a wheelchair for long distances, catheters for emptying my bladder, and supplements for my bowel movements. I couldn't accept my limited endurance and how all of my daily functional activities took significantly more time to complete than before my injury.

"I used to be able to do so much in a day. Now it takes so much effort to do what I didn't have to even think about before," I would often say with frustration and impatience. The thought of my life never returning to how it was in the past was saddening. I was also experiencing burning and shooting pain in my back, hips, ankles, and feet daily. Every time I stretched out my legs, my lower extremities would spasm into what felt like the knotting of my calves into golf balls.

"Am I really going to have to live with this for the rest of my life?" I'd ask myself often.

As daily chronic pain was beginning to unfold as a new norm for me, I started to experience more anger, fear, and grief. But with a habit of hiding emotions that I judged to be negative, I hid my emotions both from others and myself.

It took a vacation for me to realize I was feeling anxious and depressed.

A year after my accident I went to Cuba with my cousins for seven days, and instead of having sun, fun, and relaxation, I experienced sun, limitation, and irritation. Because I needed to wear ankle braces and orthotic shoes, I couldn't go into the swimming pool; I was only able to sit at the edges and dip my feet in the water. I was also frustrated with my inability to do what I most desired to do—walk on the sandy beach barefoot and go into the warm ocean.

"Will I have enough energy to walk with the group?

"Will I be in pain if I go with them?

"Will I have a place to change my catheter?" I had never had to worry about pain, fatigue, and bladder management before, and now everything I did had to be planned around these factors. Previously a carefree person, worry and anxiety were now becoming part of my daily experience.

I was also feeling a loss of my identity because the things that I identified myself with I could no longer do. For instance, I've been a dancer since I was a child. Every night my cousins would go to the club, and instead of me being in the middle of the dance floor tearing it up as always, I was either on a chair in the corner watching everyone else dance or inside my room at the hotel, lying in bed, tired.

"Just be happy that everyone else is having a good time," I would tell myself.

The all-inclusive resort we were staying at held shows each night where staff would pick volunteers from the audience to participate in whatever activity they were hosting on stage. Well, that used to be me—the enthusiastic one who would always volunteer first to get up and entertain. But not anymore—instead, the current me would be sitting down, watching in pain and fatigue or simply unable to participate in the physical tasks required on stage.

"Just be happy that everyone else is having a good time," I continued to tell myself.

Needless to say, I came back from that trip feeling confused. The expectations I had put upon myself to be happy had prevented me from acknowledging what I was really feeling inside.

"I need to go away on another trip. I need to get away and just be," I said to my mom.

So just a couple of days after I returned from Cuba, I hopped on a train and went to Ste. Anne's Spa in Grafton, Ontario, where I spent two days just being alone in silence. I had no computer, no internet, no television, no books, no music—just me, myself, my pain, nature, and God. On my second day there I joined a yoga class. Afterward, I stayed in the yoga studio to do additional stretching of my own, when a realization hit me like a truck.

"Oh my God! In the past year, not once have I stopped to honour and thank myself! To thank my mind for persevering, to thank my body for all its recovery, and to thank my soul for just being!"

After that, you can probably guess by now what I did. I journaled! I reflected on all of my milestones in the past year, and as I wrote, something came over me and words seemed to just pour out of my pen. Within an hour I had written "Celebrating Life with a Disability"—a piece that reminds us that we can acknowledge disability as a form of resistance that leads to strength. That afternoon I celebrated myself, my disability, the lessons I had learned, and the growth I'd gained.

Serendipitously, just a few days after I returned from that spa retreat I received a mass email from Spinal Cord Injury Ontario. The 2011 International Day of Persons with Disability was approaching, and they were looking for people to share their stories at Toronto City Hall. Feeling the call to share my piece, I went and I read "Celebrating Life with a Disability." After I spoke, a journalist from the *Toronto Star* approached me and asked if I could repeat my speech for them to record and share on their website.

"The *Toronto Star* website! Wow," I thought to myself. I was amazed at how I went from a state of frustration and irritation just a few weeks before to a state of inspiring others with a message of gratitude and celebration. For the next few weeks I felt great. But I later learned that positivity can only take me so far and gratitude alone is not always enough.

I Think I Am Going to Die

My favourite place to get massages in Toronto is the Elmwood Spa, because I find much benefit in using their saunas and hot tubs before getting bodywork done. One day I was sitting in a hot tub having a conversation with a girlfriend when all of a sudden my stomach felt as though it was turning into knots. Thinking I just needed a bowel movement, I went to the bathroom, but as I sat on the toilet, the knotting sensations in my belly only got worse.

"I have never felt this before. What is happening to me?" I thought to myself. "Maybe there was something in what I ate. Oh my God, am I going to die?" The pains intensified so much that they brought me to the bathroom floor, where for the next few minutes I remained hunched over, with my belly in my arms and my bathing suit bottom still around my ankles.

"I think I am going to die!" Scared for my life, I managed to crawl on my knees toward the bathroom door, opened it, and yelled for my girlfriend. "Tina! Help!"

"Oh my gosh, what's happening?" Tina said as she ran into the bathroom.

"Call for an ambulance," I said in response.

Tina used her cell phone to call for an ambulance and retrieved a staff member to help us.

Tina and one of the Elmwood staff helped me get my bathing suit bottom and robe back on. With their assistance I was able to walk over to a nearby sofa, where we waited for the paramedics to arrive. I continued to freak out as the pains seemed to get worse, until my hands started to seize up in a spasm where my fingers and wrists curled inwards so tightly they looked like lobster claws.

"What's happening to my hands?" I asked aloud in fear.

Just as I said those words, two paramedics walked through the elevator doors and headed straight toward me. As one paramedic began to take my vitals, the other looked at my clawed hands and casually said, "You're having an anxiety attack. You need to breathe."

"An anxiety attack?" I thought to myself in disbelief. I had never experienced an anxiety attack in the past and I hadn't thought I ever would.

"Why aren't they concerned about me dying?" I thought, confused by the calm and casual demeanour of the paramedics. They showed no sense of urgency.

"Am I really not dying?" I asked myself curiously. "Am I really just having an anxiety attack?" As I started to believe in the possibility that I was not dying, I started to take long deep breaths.

"Maybe I'm not dying."

To my surprise, my clawed hands began to release and relax within just a few minutes of my breathing deeply. My stomach pains also diminished.

According to the paramedics, the pains I was experiencing were probably due to my going into the hot tub without waiting long enough after I had eaten. With no apparent need to take me to the hospital, the paramedics soon left, and I spent the rest of the afternoon at the spa reflecting on what had happened.

It was humbling for me to see how quickly I can allow my mind to catastrophize, and eye-opening to learn how immediately my physical body responded to the belief "I think I am going to die" versus "maybe I'm not dying." I experienced first-hand how just the act of changing my breath from hyperventilation to long deep breaths could have a drastic impact on my body.

"I need to practise mindfulness," I realized. I had taken mindfulness classes in the past via the employee wellness program at my work, so I knew of its potential to help with pain, stress, and anxiety.

I moved forward from that anxiety attack with a stronger intention to cultivate a mindfulness practice. Unfortunately, however, not all of my healthcare providers were supportive of this practice.

He Doesn't Know Me Like I Do

Several months after that anxiety attack I returned to Sunnybrook Hospital for an assessment to be completed by an orthopaedic specialist. After he looked at my gait, reflexes, and muscle strength, I explained to him about all the various modalities I was doing, which included both traditional allopathic modalities and complementary therapies such as reflexology, acupuncture, and mindfulness.

This doctor then said to me, "The spinal cord injury has definitely impaired your balance and coordination, and I don't think that will improve significantly. All of that other stuff you're doing, the reflexology, acupuncture, yoga, meditation—none of that works. They just seem to be working for you because you believe it. But in actuality, they're not helping you."

Having been raised in a colonized culture where the white male physician is respected just for being a white male physician, I believed his words.

When I left his office and made my way back to my car, I felt some movement stirring inside my torso. Once I got inside my car and closed the driver's door, tears started to well up in my eyes. For the next twenty minutes I sat in my car crying. Believing that the doctor was right and I was so wrong, I felt like a fool for actually thinking that all the complementary modalities I was trying would help me. I felt embarrassed for being so naive, maybe desperate, and perhaps even stupid. At the same time, I started to feel overwhelmed with despair. All the complementary modalities had given me hope that I could gain more function and do more of the things that were meaningful to me. But with the efficacy of these modalities being invalidated by someone in a role that I respected, that hope diminished.

The most intimate I have gotten with the experience of despair occurred on that day when that doctor took away my hope.

Still sitting in my car, I felt lost. I felt stuck. I didn't know what to do. Much of what I had believed in had just been thrown into the garbage by someone I considered an expert in medicine. Feeling so thrown off, I couldn't even start the car, because I didn't know where to go from there. So in my confusion and desire for advice, I ended up pulling out my cell phone and doing something I hardly ever do: I journaled on Facebook! I opened up my Facebook account and wrote a post on my news feed describing what had just happened. It is probably the most vulnerable post my Facebook community has witnessed. My girlfriend Kaye Penaflor called me just minutes after I published the post.

"Jaisa, that doctor is just one person who only met you today, so he doesn't even know you. He hasn't been on your journey since day one, so he shouldn't have made those irresponsible comments not knowing how bad it was in the beginning and how far you've come! Fuck that guy. What is his name so I can call him and give him shit!" Kaye spoke with a conviction that made me start to doubt what the doctor had told me.

"Maybe I'm not so stupid then," I said. Until those moments with Kaye, my mind had been conditioned to think that doctors always know best, and thus that one doctor knew more about my body than I did.

"Jaisa, you have come so far because of the decisions you have been making! You have so many people who believe in you and support what you're doing, including myself," Kaye reminded me.

I found comfort in her words.

"He is wrong, Kaye," I realized. "And he doesn't know me like I do!"

As my belief in my decisions regarding my healing began to return, the fog of confusion lifted and I could see my future path more clearly. I believed in all of the modalities I was engaged in because I was experiencing their benefits firsthand.

"No one knows me better than I do myself," I said to Kaye with a growing tone of confidence in my voice.

After thanking Kaye and telling her that I loved her, I got off the phone, deleted my public journaling post, and turned the car on. I knew where I was going from there and I had that doctor to thank. His judgment had knocked me off from my sense of inner knowing, but in returning to myself, my confidence was strengthened. I moved forward from that day onward with a hope renewed and more drive to stay on the healing path that I create for myself.

Part II

A Way to Live in Alignment with the Reality of the Present

4

Mindfulness—the Ever-Constant Choice

The Foundational Attitudes

My anxiety attack at the Elmwood Spa was a humbling wake-up call, showing me that I needed to strengthen my ability to respond to stressful situations instead of reacting in ways that made my situation worse. I knew that I needed to cultivate more awareness and that mindfulness would be the way. So in the fall of 2012 I completed an eight-week course developed in 1979 by Jon Kabat-Zinn called Mindfulness-Based Stress Reduction (MBSR). With daily homework and a group to be accountable to each week, this course helped me to establish my own mindfulness practice.

Since that fall I have come to appreciate mindfulness as the ever-constant practice of choosing to experience the actual reality of this present moment. Until the MBSR course I thought that I was always experiencing reality, but as my awareness grew I realized that, most often, I was instead experiencing my perception of reality, an illusion of my mind.

Generally, the practice of mindfulness leads the way to an ever-expanding awareness of the true nature of things—including the nature of being human. Specifically, the practice of mindfulness helps me to align both my mind and my heart with whatever is happening in the present moment, whether it be thoughts, emotions, or sensations. I learned to do this through the cultivation of six particular attitudes described in chapter two of Kabat-Zinn's book *Full Catastrophe Living: Using the Wisdom of Your Body and Mind to Face Stress, Pain, and Illness.* According to Kabat-Zinn, non-judgment, acceptance, letting go, trust, patience, non-striving, and beginner's mind are the foundational soil upon which mindfulness is cultivated. Experiencing the true nature of each moment can arise when we set the intention to pay attention to the present moment with these foundational attitudes.

Let me give you one example of how these attitudes have helped me to experience the actual reality of some challenging moments. I was doing a mindful walk one day as part of the MBSR homework, and it was very unpleasant because I was feeling increasing pain in my feet and my back. The quality of my gait was also poor, with asymmetry between my left and right side; in common terms, I was limping. I was frustrated and angry. The pain sucked. My walking sucked. My life sucked. Five minutes into walking I realized I was supposed to bring mindfulness to the act of walking.

"Oh shit, I'm supposed to be mindful," I thought to myself. So I stopped walking and then took a moment to set the intention to let go, be curious, non-judgmental, accepting, patient, trusting, and non-striving. I then continued to walk, bringing a welcoming quality of observing to my body and whatever sensations were arising.

"My body feels tired. There's a sharp, hot pain radiating through the inside of my ankles; on a pain scale of one to ten, it feels like a five. There's a warm throbbing in my lower back that feels like a four out of ten. I feel dehydrated."

I then broadened my welcoming awareness to include whatever emotions and thoughts were arising.

"I'm having emotions of frustration and anger. I'm feeling these emotions in my neck and shoulders as tightness. I'm having thoughts of 'this pain sucks,' 'my walking sucks,' and 'my life sucks.'"

And then with just that simplicity of stepping back to gain a broader perspective of myself as both my mind and my body, an insight arose: "My life doesn't suck! I'm just having thoughts that my life sucks. And thoughts are not always fact!" In that moment I stepped out of the distorted reality that my life sucked and stepped toward alignment with actual reality.

"Oh wow. No wonder I'm tired and in pain. I've been walking this whole time without sitting down even once to rest." Finally listening to my body, I walked over to a nearby bench to sit down and rest. As I glanced down at my painful ankles, I realized I had left the house without putting on my ankle foot orthoses (AFOs), the braces that support the muscles and joints in my ankles and feet.

"Holy shit. I think I do need my AFOs. I've been in denial that I actually do need them for pain management."

So as you can see, the intention to pay attention using the foundational attitudes of mindfulness helped me to get out of my head and into my body so that I could see more clearly what actual reality called for. Let's briefly go through each attitude.

Non-judgment reminds me to see reality clearly, as it is, instead of through the filters of judgment. For instance, the thought "My walking sucks" is a judgment preventing me from experiencing my walking for how it may really be. Perhaps the quality of my walking was actually better than a month before. But if I'm stuck in my head, I can't be aware of how my perceptions may be shaping my reality.

Beginner's mind reminds me to experience the moment with the freshness and curiosity of a child experiencing something for the first time ever. As in the above example, I was able to bring curiosity to my body by acknowledging how it is always changing. The body I observe today is different from the body I observed last week. Beginner's mind also has me being curious about the mind: "How am I shaping my experience of this moment through my judgments? What is the actual reality of this moment? What is really happening here?" There is an inherent humility with beginner's mind, because it acknowledges that there is something I may not know that I don't even know! Whether the present moment is pleasant or unpleasant, this attitude of being curious leads me to ask, "What is there to be discovered here?"

Acceptance reminds me to allow the moment to be as it is even when I don't like it. I don't have to love it. I just have to acknowledge and allow the reality of the moment to be. For instance, I certainly did not like the experience of pain and fatigue, but acceptance helped me to stop resisting it and instead allowed the moment to be. After all, the sensations were already there, so to resist them would only make the experience worse. Accepting pain and fatigue doesn't mean that I have given up and given in to living this way for the rest of my life. I still have goals to improve my endurance and live pain free, but acceptance means I allow this pain and fatigue to be here, today, maybe even for the rest of this week.

Non-striving reminds me to allow myself to do nothing sometimes and to be okay with where I am in my recovery, no matter where I am on the journey. Striving to walk and run again can have me so focused on my rehab goals that I'm never happy until I reach my goal. Non-striving doesn't mean that I will no longer work hard to achieve my goals. I still continue to strive daily to get stronger. But with all the striving I do daily, non-striving simply brings balance by allowing me to take breaks and be at peace with wherever I am today.

Patience reminds me that things unfold in their own time. In the example above, I was frustrated and angry at the experience of being in pain and fatigued, and with the quality of my gait. But patience is a form of wisdom that had me listen to my body and thus stop and rest for as long as I needed. Patience reminded me that the quality of my gait will improve over time and that with rest and proper self-care, my pain and fatigue will diminish.

Trust reminds me to have faith in myself, my intuition, and my inner wisdom. Despite my limitations, I have to trust in my body and its capacity for healing, and know that there is more right with it than there is wrong. And for the moments when I'm full of self-doubt, I know I can trust in my breath to connect me with my inner resources. When all else fails, I have learned to trust in what I love, and I love the practice of mindfulness. So in the above example, I trusted that in that moment of frustration and anger, something good would come out of bringing mindfulness to the moment. And with trust like that, I continue to find motivation to stop and bring the attitudes of mindfulness to my experiences.

Finally, letting go reminds me to observe how I may be too attached to my expectations of how something should or shouldn't be. During that mindful walk, I had to finally let go of my desire to walk without AFOs. Similar to how holding onto our breath can kill us, my holding on to my need to walk without AFOs was causing my body more pain and fatigue.

Mindfulness is the ever-constant choosing to meet the

present moment with these foundational attitudes, which in turn opens the mind and heart to be in alignment with reality, even when reality presents as unpleasant or painful.

I Am Response-Able

Our ability to choose to meet the present moment mindfully rests on the truth that we are all fundamentally free. We each have the freedom to choose how we respond to life.

While I was an inpatient at TRI, I befriended another patient named John who had survived a traumatic spinal cord injury from the neck down after being thrown off his bicycle. He required a power wheelchair and maximum assistance for all his personal care, but despite this, John came to the physiotherapy gym every day with a smile on his face. His genuine smile intrigued me, so I approached him one day and said, "John, how come you're able to smile every day despite everything that's happened?"

His response: "Because I'm free. No matter what, I am still free to choose how I respond to life."

With this freedom comes the ability to respond. Indeed, we are response-able. Though this freedom is there for everyone, it is only claimed by those who choose to claim it. Mindfulness helps us to claim this freedom by creating the space for us to see reality more clearly and thus make further responses wisely instead of habitually reacting to life.

The Autopilot Mode

The difference between responding and reacting is awareness. *Responding* occurs when we are aware of the reality of the present, whereas *reacting* is like a reflex that happens automatically. When I react, I am most often re-enacting a past behaviour that I've neurally ingrained in my nervous system through habit. The more I have repeated an act, the more I easily re-enact it automatically without my conscious awareness. Reacting only occurs when I am on autopilot mode.

I actually can go through most of my day on autopilot, re-enacting every daily function. For instance, there are mornings when I'm stuck in my head, analyzing the past or planning for the future, all the while managing to bathe, dress, eat, and even commute to work. By the time I get to work, I'll often wonder, "How did I get here?"

Autopilot is actually a wonderful mechanism that our bodies utilize to remove our attention from how we carry out tasks that we often do, so that we can save energy and free up our minds to learn new tasks. The problem with autopilot arises when we spend more and more of our days in autopilot mode instead of awareness mode, reacting more than responding. Imagine that you have a car that has an autopilot mode button. If you were to put the car on autopilot mode, who would be in control of the car? The car? Or you? The car. Similarly, if you were going about your day on autopilot mode, it would not be you who was in conscious control of the day's experiences but your body just re-enacting wired behaviours like a robot.

The Cow Path

I myself found much comfort when I learned that I wasn't the only one who lived on autopilot. As I learned more about the MBSR program, I discovered the term "cow path," which many mindfulness teachers actually use to demonstrate how we humans have habits of reacting to stress that are inefficient and thus unhealthy. Picture a cow taking a long, roundabout, winding way to get from point A to point B. While the path (which is well trodden) is clearly not energy efficient, the cow takes the path simply because of habit. So just as cows tread a path in the grass with repeated use, we humans tread neural paths in our brains with the repetition of our habits.

Awareness Trumps Habit

I find even more comfort in remembering this: awareness always trumps habit, and we are more than the sum of our habits. If we think of the neurally wired body as a computer, we can also think of our awareness as the programmer of the computer. No matter how densely wired a computer program is, the programmer always trumps the computer. So whenever I find myself operating on autopilot, I simply remind myself that my awareness trumps habit.

Whether we bring attention to the breath, our feet, the food we are eating, or the visual scene in front of us, stepping out of autopilot mode is as easy as bringing our attention back to something that is happening in real time, in the moment.

Going back to the example of my mindful walk, it was through the intention of paying attention to the moment with the foundational attitudes of mindfulness that I was able to move from feeling frustrated and angry to feeling a sense of empowerment and control through my sense of response-ability. In acknowledging the actual reality of my needs, I gained understanding and insight and was able to create a plan for minimizing the onset of future pain. That involved listening to my body better, slowing down, and resting when needed, and though I didn't like it, I came to accept wearing AFOs.

5

Responding to the Body

Paying Attention Does Pay Out

"How does that feel?" my physiotherapists would often ask.

"Uh, I don't know," I'd often reply.

"How does this feel now in comparison to before?" they'd ask after performing a modality.

"I can't recall. I wasn't paying attention." Actually I was always paying attention—just not to my body. Instead, I paid attention to what the people around me were doing, what was on the television, or most often I was paying attention to my thoughts.

I've now taken the MBSR course twice as a participant, and both times the most challenging practice for me has been the body scan—a meditation in which one scans the entire body with mindful attention. With many years spent living in my head, I had unknowingly developed a habit of ignoring my body and its needs. For instance, as part of the daily homework for the MBSR course, I had to pay attention to the thoughts, emotions, and bodily sensations I was experiencing, in other words, the mind and the body. Over time I began to see my pattern of saying "later" to my body.

I would be so attached to the goals and plans I had set

in my mind that if my body was hungry or thirsty, I'd say to myself, "Later, after this task is done."

If my body wanted to go to the washroom, I'd say to myself, "Later, after this task is done."

And if my body was in pain and needed rest or care, you guessed it: I'd say to myself, "Later, after this task is done."

Waking up to the reality that I was living outside my body instead of within it inspired me to pay more attention to my body—not just any kind of attention but attention that is non-judgmental, accepting, curious, patient, trusting, and non-striving. As I later discovered, paying attention in these particular ways does in fact pay out!

In January 2012 I signed up for a ten-day Vipassana retreat (as taught by S. N. Goenka). This is a guided meditation retreat where, other than during the teacher's discourse each night and the few occasions when retreatants can ask the teacher questions, the majority of the ten days is spent paying attention to the body via forty-five-minute body scans multiple times a day.

Having read some of Jon Kabat-Zinn's articles, I recognized that one of his teachings was prominent in my mind during this retreat. It was his reinterpreting of the term "rehabilitation" as a way of reinhabiting one's body as it is right now in the present moment As a therapist who worked in rehabilitation, for me this term had always brought with it an underlying intention to get someone back to the way they were prior to injury or illness. But now that I have experienced being a patient, this intention represents for me a desperate sense of striving to get back to the way someone was before their injury, with little focus on accepting their body as it is now. So, in just the way one would excitedly reinhabit a newly renovated home, for the duration of the retreat, whether I was sitting, lying down, standing, walking, bathing, dressing, or eating, I curiously reinhabited every inch of my body.

A few days after returning from that retreat, I went to see my physiotherapist Kyle Whaley for our regular weekly session. When I walked into his clinic, Kyle glanced my way, and as soon as he saw me walking he said, "Hey! Wow, what did you do there?" Apparently my gait had significantly improved.

"I didn't do anything. I didn't even do any of my exercises. I just paid attention to my body," I replied.

In one of Jon Kabat-Zinn's earlier yet groundbreaking studies, he looked at the effects of meditation on the skin disease psoriasis.[1] The study had two groups. Both groups of participants with psoriasis received ultraviolet (UV) light treatment. However, one group was to meditate and pay attention to their breath while inside the UV light machine. Even though both groups received the same light treatment, the group that meditated experienced significantly more improvement in the clearing of their psoriasis symptoms than the non-meditating group. Scientists and clinicians commonly refer to this study, because it clearly demonstrates the mind-body connection and how just paying attention with the mind causes something to happen to the body.

Fewer Cues Needed

The simple act of paying more attention to my body also contributed to my recovery, because in paying better attention, I required fewer cues from my therapists. If you don't have a physical limitation, you probably don't require cues to remind you how to move efficiently, but when I first learned to stand up from a seated position, I required the daily reminder from my therapists to pay attention to how my feet were on the ground, where to place my hands, how to keep my shoulders back, how to shift my weight forward to stand, and how to engage my core and buttocks.

Of course, with practice and thanks to neuroplasticity, most activities can be relearned and fewer external cues required over time. But for me, practising only in the physio gym was not enough. I wanted to practise as much as I could, and that's how a daily mindfulness practice helped me. With growing awareness of my body and how it moved in each moment, I was able to make any functional activity a therapeutic session. Instead of just practising sit-to-stands when I was in physiotherapy, I practised standing up from sitting on the bed, the sofa, a car, the dining room chair, and the toilet, engaging my body in the ways my therapists always cued. Moments that would have otherwise been mundane moments became therapeutic moments because of mindfulness.

Unlearning Compensatory Strategies

Paying more attention to my body also has helped me to unlearn compensatory strategies, a term referring to the ways in which the body compensates for a weakness or deficit. Our bodies are efficient and thus will take the easiest route to complete tasks. So if my body had the option to use my arms to push and/or pull myself up to standing, versus going through the painful effort to re-engage my feet, legs, buttocks, and core to stand up, my body would compensate and choose the easier route.

It is important to note here that when I am not aware of myself, the body takes the easy route, meaning my body often compensates when I'm not paying attention. For instance, whenever I walked with my canes without awareness, I would automatically lean on the canes, using my upper body strength to bear the weight of my body. But when I was aware of my body, I would remember to engage my lower extremities and bear weight through them instead, leading to an improvement in the quality of my gait over time. With less time practising compensation and more time practising quality movement, mindfulness continues to contribute to my recovery and my return to maximal function.

A Relationship with Pain

In paying more attention to my body, I have become more aware of its sensations, and that includes the painful sensations too. That's because mindfulness does not discriminate what it pays attention to; it is merely a practice. Whether I am experiencing sensations that are pleasant or unpleasant, mindfulness reminds me to pay attention with the same quality of an open mind and an open heart.

Prior to taking the MBSR course I used to ignore my chronic pain, thinking that somehow distracting myself from feeling it would make the pain go away. During the times when I couldn't ignore the pain, I thought that I could just endure it with grit. But now that I've lived with chronic pain for over seven years, I know that ignoring and enduring pain can only take me so far. If I'm going to continue to live well with pain, I have to maintain a mindful relationship with pain.

With the foundational attitudes of mindfulness I have been able to develop a healthy relationship with pain. The practice of acceptance and non-judgment helps me at the very least to acknowledge the reality of what I'm feeling. Trust reminds me that pain is often communicating something and that just as it arose, it will also pass, which then encourages me to be patient. But the attitude that has helped me the most in developing a working relationship with pain is beginner's mind.

"What are the qualities of this pain?

"On of a scale of zero to ten, where zero means no pain and ten is the most intense pain I've experienced, how would I describe my pain?

"What message does this pain have for me?

"How can I take better care of myself today? What do I need to do to nourish myself?"

Instead of ignoring or trying to endure pain, asking myself these types of curious questions has helped me to turn toward pain, facing it with hope that there may be something I can gain.

Turning toward the Pain = Gain

In the last chapter I gave an example of how turning toward the pain led to the understanding that I needed to rest, slow down, and wear my AFOs. In the continued practice of paying attention to chronic pain, I've also learned that if I don't drink enough water or if I eat too much gluten and dairy (I'm sensitive to both), my muscles will feel sore and stiff later that day. If I don't do my daily yoga for stretching and strengthening, and get outdoors for fresh air at least once a day, I'll feel tired, heavy, and stiff throughout my body and have more pain in my feet and back. Lastly, if I'm feeling stressed, depressed, or anxious, then whatever pain I'm feeling is intensified with my emotions.

In addition to the understanding and insight that arises from paying attention to pain is the sense of courage and control that arises in my choosing to turn toward the pain. With every instance that I exert my freedom to choose to meet pain mindfully instead of choosing to judge and resist it, my sense of fear and lack of control in the face of pain diminishes.

But the most important thing that I continue to gain from being in a relationship with pain is the decrease in pain intensity over the years. I used to experience pain of anywhere from four to six out of ten at least once a month. But in the last few years I've only experienced that intensity of pain two to three times a year. Of course, new pains arise here and there as my body continues to recover. But the intensity and, more importantly, the functional impacts pain has on my life have decreased over time with the help of a mindfulness practice as a complement to my other therapies.

One person whose work has inspired me to shape my experience of pain by how I relate to it is physiotherapist and yoga therapist Neil Pearson. His work, which he offers through Life Is Now Pain Care™, has helped both professionals and patients to better understand the neurophysiology of the pain experience, consequently motivating us to not only cope better with pain but eventually even decrease our pain.

On his website Pain Care for Life (lifeisnow.ca), Neil offers research-based education on pain neurophysiology and pain management. One resource that I often refer to is the educational e-book *Understand Pain, Live Well Again*, authored by Neil in 2008.[2] This is a valuable resource available online for free via the "First 5 Steps" link on his home page. In this ebook, Neil describes how we can experience signals from our physical body on a continuum between "dangerous" and "not dangerous." Our conscious interpretation of the pain will then moderate how we continue to experience the pain. When we perceive the problem as "really dangerous," then the brain will send messages to the nerves in our spinal cord, leading to an increase in the actual danger signals coming to the brain.

Consequently, we will actually experience more pain.

If the brain were the president of the body and it decided that a pain experience or a danger signal was a significant threat to the body, it would tell the nerves in the spinal cord, "Hey, guys, we are under attack. Let's raise the threat alert from green to red and be on the lookout. Let me know anything that has to do with this threat." In response, the nerves in the spinal cord would be more sensitive to danger signals and relay even more signals, meaning we might experience more pain.

However, if the brain perceives the signal as "not dangerous," then messages are sent to the spinal cord to either block or decrease signals from the body. For instance, back to the above metaphor, if the brain were president and knew that the signals were not a threat but merely a temporary experience, it would tell the spinal cord, "Hey, guys, I know these stimuli are not a threat to us, so don't even bother telling me about it. I have other things to do." Consequently, we will actually experience less pain.

Reflecting back on my anxiety attack at the Elmwood Spa, when I believed my thought "I think I'm going to die," I equate that to both my brain perceiving the stimuli as "really dangerous" and my consciousness believing that this was truth. This then led to my pain getting worse. But as soon as I realized that I was not dying, my perception changed to "not dangerous" and the pain quickly subsided.

Depending on my relationship with pain, I will lean toward perceiving painful sensations as either "really dangerous" or "not dangerous." For instance, when I have a fearful relationship with pain, I'm more likely to have perceptions of "really dangerous," with thoughts such as "I can't handle this; this is too much; life sucks; I'm getting worse." Whereas if I'm in a mindful relationship with pain, I'm more likely to have perceptions that are "not dangerous," with thoughts such as "Hmm, I wonder what this pain is telling me; maybe I'm dehydrated; this sensation is temporary and will pass; I can be with this moment."

Supporting my experience of using mindfulness to cope with pain is a growing body of scientific evidence demonstrating how mindfulness correlates with increases in non-reactivity (the ability to respond versus react), the reinterpretation of pain sensations, and the positive reappraisal of pain. All these help us to relate to pain with more openness. Mindfulness has also been found to correlate with decreases in pain sensitivity, opioid craving and misuse, and pain-attentional bias (meaning people learn to focus less on pain). One of my favourite findings, though, is the data supporting the correlation between mindfulness and a decrease in pain-related functional interference; in other words, mindfulness can help with our return to engaging in daily functional activities.[3]

I personally find hope and enthusiasm in the fact that not only are we free to choose to be in a relationship with pain or not but also a growing body of science shows how the courageous act of relating to pain mindfully can lead to both a decrease in pain and an increase in our resiliency and ability to live well with pain.

6

Too Busy to Be Real

Becoming a Mindless Mindfulness Teacher

While I've been able to be in relationship with my physical pains, I have found it more challenging to acknowledge emotional pains. Perhaps it is because chronic pain only arose in my life when I was thirty years old, so developing new habits of relating to physical pain was easier. Whereas with emotional pains, these are experiences that I've habitually yet unknowingly ignored since I was a child, leaving me with the task of unlearning old patterns in the midst of learning new patterns of relating to emotional pain. Throughout my teens and twenties I distracted myself from uncomfortable emotions by keeping myself busy. That was my cow path. So after the accident I remained on that cow path and kept myself busy with rehab and eventually mindfulness work.

Inspired by the MBSR program and its potential to help people, I went on to pursue training at the Center for Mindfulness at the University of Massachusetts Medical School (now called the Oasis Institute). There I completed the seven-day Professional Training, the nine-day Intensive Practicum, and the eight-day Teacher Development Intensive in MBSR.

As a qualified MBSR teacher with an enthusiasm to share

the benefits of mindfulness, I returned to work in the fall of 2012, just thirteen months after my accident. By 2015 I had taught over twenty cycles of the MBSR program to patients experiencing stress, anxiety, depression, and chronic pain. I provided mindfulness education at rehabilitation hospitals, psychiatry clinics, wellness centres, conferences, high schools, and universities. I also provided MBSR on a one-on-one basis to patients with brain injuries who needed personal modifications to the program. My rehab team was of the greatest support to me, not only asking me to teach mindfulness to their colleagues but referring their patients to me as well.

What a blessing to have many patients being referred to me. However, with no prior experience in being self-employed and a long habit of people pleasing, I did not know how to create healthy boundaries. I said yes to almost every referral that came to me, even if it meant seeing more clients than I had time for, driving longer distances than I should have, and overextending myself to do more MBSR cycles than my body could handle. Throughout 2012–15, I got busier and busier teaching mindfulness, so that by 2015 I had put my own rehabilitation on the back burner.

Preaching more than practising, I was becoming a mindless mindfulness teacher.

Jaisa, You Need to Slow Down

"You need to get off the highway," my shiatsu healer insisted.

"I know I need to slow down," I replied.

But knowing is one thing and realizing is another. I didn't understand the imperativeness of my slowing down my pace of life until a few incidents occurred in 2015.

I was driving home one night and was just a few seconds

before driving onto the on-ramp to Ontario Highway 401 when a cop pulled up behind me and signalled for me to pull over. I was confused because I was not speeding and couldn't think of any reason why I'd be pulled over. The police officer ended up doing a check on my driver's license and license plate. When I asked him what I had done wrong, he replied, "Nothing. Just a random stop."

After the cop drove off, I sat in my car for a few moments feeling confused.

"What was that all about?" I thought to myself.

Perplexed, I looked up at the night sky and asked the universe, "What is the meaning of this?"

I curiously listened for an answer. And then it happened. The words "get off the highway" arose in my mind.

"Hmm. Wow. That's interesting," I thought to myself. "A cop pulls me over before I get on the highway."

Whether it was a divine message reminding me to slow down or just a random event that I didn't need to read into, I decided to play it safe and took note of the nudge to slow down.

Several weeks after that night I was in my car on my way to see a client when I had another "you need to slow down" moment. As I pulled out of the driveway of my townhome, I fortunately took a moment to bring awareness to myself. When I realized what I was doing, I thought, "Jaisa, what the fuck?"

I had one hand on the driving wheel, the other hand was holding a slice of pizza, and in my ears were my earbuds with the microphone by my mouth so that I could compose an email via voice-to-text—all while driving. Prior to that moment, I used to pride myself on my ability to multitask. But right then and there, I realized that my ability to multitask was going to lead to my death one day.

The last straw to my fast-paced life happened while I was visiting my partner TJ in Vancouver for my thirty-sixth birthday. It was my last night with him, and so he had made me a special dinner.

But I had work to do.

I had booked a studio for my return to Toronto so that I could record my first compilation of guided mindfulness audio, so I was up late in Vancouver working on my scripts. By the time I finished, it was almost eleven at night. I looked over into the living room and my heart dropped. TJ had fallen asleep on the floor waiting for me. The dinner he had prepared for us was uneaten and cold.

"Jaisa, you need to slow down," I said to myself.

In those moments I woke up to how my speed of life had disabled my ability to prioritize what was meaningful to me. I woke up the next day with a clear decision—I was going to leave my fast-paced hustling life in Toronto and move to Vancouver with the intention to take a one-year sabbatical, slow down, and refocus on my healing.

I Create My Own Suffering

Paving the way for me to face the painful realities of life was a course that I had "mistakenly" registered for. The late Michael Stone, founder of the Centre of Gravity in Toronto, was hosting a six-day Intensive in Contemplative Care Training provided by the New York Zen Center for Contemplative Care (NYZCCC). I got a few occupational therapists to register with me, telling them, "This will be a great way for us to learn how to have more compassion for our patients!" I was not aware that for the duration of the six days I would be exploring my own suffering and learning how I was the one creating it. Had I known these were the learning objectives of the course, I probably would not have registered. But I soon understood that, since compassion is the desire for suffering to be relieved, I actually can't have compassion for myself if I first don't acknowledge that I am suffering. My capacity to create compassionate space for myself when I'm suffering the most is the extent to which I can hold compassionate space for others when they're suffering.

Our teachers were the founders and co-executive directors of the NYZCCC—Sensei Robert Chodo Campbell and Sensei Koshin Paley Ellison. Both skillfully led the group through exercises done in a large group, a small group, triads, pairs, and solos. But the most powerful exercise that I took away from that course is an exploration done in pairs and centred around one question: "How do you create your own suffering?"

My partner and I had decided I would go first. She asked, "Jaisa, how do you create your own suffering?"

"I create my own suffering by setting unrealistic expectations for myself and then beating myself up when I don't achieve them. And when I do accomplish things, I either don't take credit for them or I don't take time to celebrate myself," I responded.

"Thank you," my partner said. "Jaisa, how else do you create your own suffering?"

"I create my own suffering by not listening to my body whenever it tells me to drink more water or even when it tells me to stop and rest," I said.

"Thank you. Jaisa, how else do you create your own suffering?" she said again.

"I create my own suffering by not expressing what I really think and how I feel, because I worry about what others will think of me. I please others at the expense of pleasing myself."

"Thank you. Jaisa, how else do you create your own suffering?" she said.

"I create my own suffering by taking responsibility for how other people feel. I feel like it's my responsibility to make others happy, and if they are disappointed I put the blame on myself."

"Thank you. Jaisa, how else do you create your own suffering?"

This back and forth questioning and responding went for five to seven minutes, after which my partner and I switched roles so that I then asked her how she created her own suffering. After she had her five to seven minutes of answering the same question, we switched roles again so I had another chance to go deeper into exploring how I created my own suffering. Finally we switched roles again and my partner got to have her second chance to deepen her understanding of her role in her suffering.

Repeating the phrase "I create my own suffering by" over and over forced me to reflect on how I was treating myself. But hearing my partner also share how she created her own suffering in similar ways showed me our common humanity. I found such comfort in learning that my habits of self-judgment and self-sabotage were not unique to me.

"What a relief to know we are not alone in our self-torture!" I told my partner. We then laughed at ourselves for a little bit.

This "I create my own suffering" exercise was transformative and empowering, leaving my partner and me with more clarity on how we could better take care of ourselves. I've gone on to share this activity with early childhood educators, social workers, nurses, occupational therapists, physical therapists, and other body workers, and the common feedback I have received is that this exploration brings about a sense of ownership for our lives. The words "I create" wake us up to the reality that, just as we are response-able for the creation of our suffering, we are response-able for the creation of our compassionate self-care, healing, and wellness.

So humane is this self-imposition of suffering that the Buddha addresses it in one of his teachings, called the Sallatha Sutta, in which he describes two arrows. The first arrow represents the physical and emotional pains that naturally come with being human. The second arrow, however, refers to how we react to these pains with resistance, such as the times when I ignore my chronic pain or uncomfortable feelings of grief, fear, and anger. Whether I'm conscious of it or not, resisting pain is actually a choice I make. This means I am actually the one response-able for shooting the second arrow at myself. In this sense, we can see how "shooting the second arrow" is another term for how I create my own suffering. The take-home message for many who are inspired by this story of the two arrows is that while pain is inevitable, suffering is an option.

Mindfulness helps me to meet the first arrow (emotional and physical pain) with curious acceptance, thus helping me to stop shooting the second arrow at myself. Furthermore, in gaining understanding and insight from meeting pain mindfully, I am better able to discern when I can (or cannot) change the first arrow. For instance, in getting to know my chronic pain, fatigue, grief, fear, and anger better, I've learned that getting outside and connecting with the earth's elements decreases the intensity of these physical and emotional feelings. As a result, I try to engage with nature daily, which results in a decrease in the frequency and/or intensity of these feelings. In other words, mindfulness not only helps me to stop shooting second arrows at myself but it also affects life's first arrows. And since how I feel affects those around me, the best part about shooting fewer arrows at myself is that they're less likely to hit and harm those around me as well.

7

When Reality Is Too Painful to Face

Allowing Pain to Carve My Vessel

In the summer of 2015 I moved to Vancouver with the intention to slow down and refocus on my healing full time. Curious to explore the effects of taking my rehabilitation into the natural environment, TJ and I found an apartment on Beach Avenue in the downtown West End neighbourhood. Before the move, I was commuting for one to two hours on weekends to go to the beaches in Toronto just so that I could practise walking on the sand barefoot. Walking on sand was the only time I could walk therapeutically without shoes and orthotics, because with every step the sand forms an instant orthotic. From our new home in Vancouver, getting to the beach required only a thirty-second walk; Stanley Park was a five-minute bike ride away, and the mountains covered with temperate rainforests were only a twenty-minute drive away.

Though the quick access to nature later proved to be beneficial for my wellness, my first couple of months in Vancouver were full of suffering. Perhaps it was because I went from one extreme to another: from working full time and having too much to do each day to no job and nothing to do. With no clients to see and no workshops to teach, I found myself sleeping in each day, unmotivated to get out of bed. I was growing in irritability and would take out my moodiness on TJ. The grey rainy weather that is typical of Vancouver's fall and winter seasons also didn't help.

I did not know how to not be busy.

With less busyness keeping me occupied, I was becoming more aware of my emotions of fear, worry, anger, and sadness. I was not comfortable with these emotions, so at first I distracted myself from facing them by smoking a lot of marijuana every day, taking long afternoon naps, and watching movies or a network series every night.

I was also feeling guilty for taking the time off work to focus on my healing. But that quickly changed when I attended a workshop facilitated by a traditional herbalist and medicine keeper named Angela Angel.

"When you don't heal yourself first, you become a disservice to those you serve," Angela said.

Her words landed deeply, helping me to move forward with a renewed sense of purpose to serve myself guilt-free. To think that I'm being selfish in focusing on my healing is to forget that I am worthy of my own compassion. For the next few months, not only did I stop feeling guilty for taking the time to take care of myself, but I also began to read through all of my journals that I had kept since I was twelve years old. They were inspiring but also uncomfortable for me to read. I was inspired to see how grateful and faithful I was, but I was also saddened to see more clearly how I had been suffering from chronic self-judgment for two decades. It was painful to look back and see how I'd had little sense of who I really was. Consequently, I hadn't been able to really love or trust myself, and so I often wrote about being jealous, insecure, doubtful, and confused.

I've heard some say that mindfulness is not for the meek and I agree, because mindfulness has led me to acknowledge all of my experiences, both the joys and the pains. There were many days when reading through my journals would make me feel scared.

I wrote this in my journal on one of those grey rainy days.

Oh God. I do want to escape this suffering of being human but I cannot escape this body and mind. With compassionate awareness I can embrace and hold the pain, accepting it and integrating it all.

Being new to the experience of sitting with my emotional pains, I had to psych myself up somehow. Inspired by Kahlil Gibran's *The Prophet* and Joyce Rupp's *The Cup of Our Life* — where pain is referred to as that which carves our cups, allowing them to hold more joy—I thought of my body as a vessel, a vessel that I could allow pain to carve. Just as we can carve a wooden cup with a knife, both physical and emotional pains can feel like a knife carving into the vessel of our body. Though the carving can hurt, I find purpose in knowing that 1) the more carving I am brave enough to feel, the deeper the vessel of who I am becomes and 2) the deeper my vessel, the more of life's pains and joys I can hold for both myself and others.

The Lie of My Conditional Worth

In the welcoming of pain to carve my vessel, I have been able to face the scarier corners of my being. It was there in the shadows of my unconscious beliefs that I discovered a specific lie that has been preventing me from living in alignment with the truth that I am unconditionally worthy of my own compassion.

On one of those grey rainy days in the fall of 2015, I woke up and was immediately at war with myself. "I slept for nine hours! I'm so lazy," I thought to myself. I hadn't even gotten out of bed yet, and already my day was not going according to plan. I lay in bed for another half hour feeling unmotivated to do anything, until another thought came: "Let's face this. After all, I came here to heal!" I then rolled over to reach my journal on my nightstand and began to write with curiosity.

Observing the thoughts that were unfolding onto the pages of my journal, I started to sense the harsh judgmental critic in me. Thoughts of "I shouldn't have slept so long; I have no discipline; I haven't accomplished anything this week; I should be doing more; she's better than me; I'm better than him" came to mind.

As I looked at the words reflecting the state of my mind, I expanded my awareness to include my emotions and sensations. I was angry, anxious, and disappointed. I felt tight, blocked, and heavy. With the intention to be non-judgmental and accepting, I welcomed how I was feeling, until all of a sudden I started to cry.

"Where is this coming from?" I wondered with interest. Allowing myself the opportunity to feel how I was feeling, I cried for several more minutes. Oddly, it was feeling good to just cry. As the last few tears continued to roll down my face, I meditated, continuing to create accepting, curious space for myself to just be. As if out of nowhere, an insight suddenly arose and I discovered an underlying belief that I never even knew I held.

"My worth is conditional!"

As I realized this, my world in that moment began to open up and I began to see with more clarity how I was living my life according to this lie.

"Oh my God. My sense of worthiness, my belief that I am worthy of my own love, compassion, and respect, is conditional upon my ability to accomplish, succeed, achieve, and be productive. If I do not tick off everything on the unrealistic to-do list that I made for myself, then I judge myself." The light of my growing awareness started to shine on the extent of my chronic self-judgment.

"My sense of worth is also conditional upon being right, being better, knowing more than others, and being well liked. If these conditions are not met, then I judge myself!" Though it was painful to face the harmful ways of my own ego, the clarity that came in seeing this reality was liberating.

"I stress myself out in my effort to be accomplished, I get anxious in my need to be productive or be the best, and I get depressed when I don't accomplish, produce, or end up being the best." My role in the creation of my own mental illness was now apparent.

"No wonder I've been struggling with myself here in Vancouver. I am an overachiever and for the first time in decades I am no longer busy doing the things that give me a sense of worth. The belief that 'I am only worthy when …' is the driving force that has me going past my body's limits, ignoring its needs, all in the pursuit of doing, doing, doing. For it is in the doing, not the being, that I judge myself worthy of my own love."

For a few minutes I felt anger. I was mad at myself for the suffering I had put myself through for so long. Mindfully allowing myself to be angry, I soon began to understand that my anger was a direct reflection of my compassion for myself.

"Wow. I'm angry because I love myself! I've never felt this kind of compassion for myself!" I thought. I liked how this new way of being in relation to myself felt, so I made a promise to myself. I looked out the window and gazed at the mountains before me. With Cypress Mountain, Grouse Mountain, and Mount Seymour bearing witness, I proclaimed: "From this moment onward, my sense of worthiness is unconditional! No matter what I do or don't do, how bad or how good I am, how much I know or how little I know, I am always unconditionally worthy of my own love, compassion, and respect. I am unconditionally worthy!"

Since that promise, while I still do notice self-judgmental thoughts arising, because of a consistent mindfulness practice and neuroplasticity, I am observing a decrease in the frequency of self-judgmental thoughts arising. When judgmental thoughts do arise, I am finding it easier to be in a friendly relationship with the ego, as judgmental as it can be. Whenever I notice judgmental thoughts, I am now able to befriend them the way Vietnamese mindfulness teacher Thich Nhat Hanh commonly encourages throughout his teachings. I smile at the thoughts and say, "Hello, judgment. Hello, self-loathing. You're back! I see you and I know you very well."

While my ego still gets the best of me and I forget to be kind to myself at times, relative to one year ago, two years ago, three years ago, and so on, I don't get caught in the pattern of judgment as often. Now, if I am limited by pain or fatigue and I am only able to do half the things I planned to do on a particular day, I know I am enough. My worthiness is no longer conditional upon the amount of things I do, how I do them, and whether I'm better or worse than others. My worthiness is now inherent in simply being alive.

Self-Esteem versus Self-Compassion

Some have told me that I am courageous to be so open about

my experiences of self-judgment, but actually I am not. I am honest simply because I know that my lack of self-compassion is not unique to me.

In the spring of 2014, I was in Massachusetts for the Twelfth Annual International Scientific Conference for Clinicians, Researchers, and Educators: Investigating and Integrating Mindfulness in Medicine, Health Care, and Society. I had the opportunity to listen to Kristin Neff, PhD, one of the leading researchers on self-compassion. Dr. Neff's presentation was called "Self-Compassion, Psychological Wellbeing, and the Relief of Suffering." Hearing Dr. Neff's presentation reminded me that I was not alone in my lack of self-compassion.

One insight that stood out for me during her talk was the difference between self-esteem and self-compassion. According to Dr. Neff, self-esteem is a sense of feeling good that comes in being better than others. She shared the problems with self-esteem, such as narcissism, ego-defensiveness, and the social comparison that arises from the need to be above average, which is impossible considering everyone can't be better than everyone else.

I can personally vouch for the unhealthiness in growing up with more focus on self-esteem than on self-compassion. With my worth conditional upon being more successful than others, I was always comparing myself to others. My need to be better than others has been a driving force in my overachieving and perfectionist behaviours, ultimately leading to my anxieties and depressions. The focus on self-esteem over self-compassion also fueled my self-limiting and self-sabotaging behaviours because every time I heard of someone else who was successful in a project or a field that I wanted to pursue, I discouraged myself with thoughts of "she's already at the top so I won't even bother trying."

In the past whenever I found myself falling into a depression, I would try to make myself feel better by listing everything positive about myself. But this only gave me temporary relief, serving as a band-aid solution, because as soon as I became aware of my human weaknesses I would fall back into self-judgmental patterns. According to Dr. Neff, self-compassion is about self-acceptance and not so much about self-improvement. It is about relating to myself kindly, rather than relating to myself positively. No wonder many of the self-help books that I'd read throughout my teens and twenties never really helped me. In all my efforts to change, grow, and be better I never stopped to accept myself in all my human traits, simply as I was.

We are fortunate to live in a time when there is now the science to support not only mindfulness but self-compassion as well. Dr. Neff herself has completed a vast amount of research demonstrating how self-compassion can lead to enhanced motivation and wellbeing; healthier behaviours, such as decreased substance abuse, increased physical activity; healthier body image; greater personal accountability; enhanced other-focused concerns, such as abilities to forgive and empathize; better romantic relationships; and finally, greater resiliency, as exhibited by decreased depression, anxiety, and stress, and improved immune function.[4]

A Trance State

Just as I now know that my chronic self-judgment is not unique to me, I also know that I am not the only one who gets pulled into the lie that my worth is conditional. Psychologist and meditation teacher Tara Brach actually describes the belief in our unworthiness as a trance. I love that she calls it as it is, because the reality is that we are all unconditionally worthy, and so to believe otherwise can only occur when we are in a trance state.

Some of the darkest periods in my life were actually when I was living in a trance state, caught in the belief that my worthiness was dependent upon a partner loving me. Throughout my twenties, I dated like a monkey swinging from branch to branch, only letting go of one partner when I already had the other hand holding on to the next. Lacking unconditional love for myself, I had an inner void that no one's love could ever fill. I eventually cheated on one of my partners with a stranger that I met while travelling Europe. I soon broke up with my partner and made plans to move to Europe, where I was to convert to the religion of the stranger I had met and live on a farm with him and his family. To think, I made all those plans based on just a handful of days with someone I barely even knew!

But the craziest trance I've ever been in was when I tried to get myself pregnant so that my partner at the time would not leave me. As embarrassing as it is for me to admit the intention I had for bringing a child into this world, it is the ugly truth of what the lie of unworthiness can do to someone. Unworthiness is a trance that can have us do crazy things. Fortunately, I've learned with practice over time that awareness always trumps the ego. As long as I continue to cultivate mindfulness and compassion, I find it getting easier and easier to free myself from the trance and realign myself to the truth that I am always worthy of my love.

Scrooge Moments

Whenever I wake up from the autopilot mode of trance state,

I always discover something about myself. Sometimes I learn of great things, such as how creative, wise, and compassionate I can be. Other times I learn of not so great things, such as how I have been inflicting pain on others and myself. I call the discovery of these not so great moments "Scrooge moments."

In Charles Dickens's *A Christmas Carol*, Ebenezer Scrooge—with the help of three ghosts—wakes up not only to his own childhood pains but also to the pains that he has put upon others. But in his awakening to his unconscious ways of being, he begins on a path of reconciliation. So in light of the healing Scrooge went through, I use the term "Scrooge moments" to describe when I wake up to my unconscious habits of causing harm to both myself and to others.

I think that we all experience Scrooge moments, and I think it's a normal part of our growth as humans. Initially it was hard for me to accept this harmful aspect of my nature, but like Scrooge, waking up to the bite of reality can lead to growth and transformation. For instance, a very common Scrooge moment for me is whenever I realize that I am blaming someone else for something that is my responsibility. I have blamed my mom, my dad, my partners, my friends, my co-workers, my culture, society, and I've even blamed God. While it is hard to admit this habit, it is in accepting and getting to know this habit of blaming others that I have learned how the act of blaming actually is an act of releasing my power to the one(s) whom I blame. In claiming responsibility for my role in situations, I am then also reclaiming my power.

Another example of a Scrooge moment that led to my healing and growth was when I was on Facebook one day and saw the post of a colleague who was being acknowledged for her contributions to our community. I was surprised. Observing my surprise, I then felt some guilt.

"What's going on here?" I thought to myself. Open to discovering something new about myself, I pulled out my journal and wrote:

> *January 24, 2018*
> *I have been finding my comfort in the belief that I am better than her. This belief was like a veil preventing me from acknowledging the reality of who she really is, a compassionate, wise, and humble person. So when I realized the powerful person she is and work she does I was embarrassed, because in my need to be better than others I chose to live according to my perceived reality that I am better. Living in the delusional bubble of my mind has closed me off to the abundance around me in the form of amazing people and a community who makes the present and the future brighter.*

The journey of self-awareness has led me to both the lightest and the darkest parts of myself. But unlike Ebenezer Scrooge, I didn't get to have three ghosts to help me look into the mirror clearly. What I did have and continue to have is the ability to bring mindfulness and compassion to my experiences. We all have this ability. While it can be scary to look at what the mirror reflects back to us, especially when it shows how we may be the cause of suffering for others and our own selves, Scrooge moments are always opportunities.

In my first example of a Scrooge moment, I was able to turn my pattern of blaming into a new habit of reclaiming my power. In the second example, I was able to turn my need to be better than others into a new habit of acknowledging the gifts others have to offer, and consequently my world became more abundant. Scrooge moments have been opportunities for me to discover and understand more about myself and bring healing through the acknowledgment and integration of parts of myself I previously judged and ignored. Scrooge moments provide a platform for me to understand, forgive, and accept myself, which over time has been transforming my chronic self-judgment into new patterns of unconditional self-love.

Mindfulness and Self-Compassion

Just as there is research that supports mindfulness and self-compassion, there is also research supporting the benefits of both mindfulness and self-compassion together. Research shows that when mindfulness and self-compassion are practised together, results can include a reduction in stress, an enhancement of wellbeing, and a promotion of resilience.[5]

Where mindfulness helps me to curiously open my heart and mind to experience the reality of the present moment, self-compassion motivates me to accept and fully feel the moment—whether it is pleasant or unpleasant—so that I can stop the suffering that comes with resisting life's moments. Where mindfulness helps me to acknowledge when I am experiencing pain and suffering, compassion fuels me to respond in ways that ease my pain and suffering.

When practised together, mindfulness and self-compassion have helped me to move out of the bubble of my judgmental mind and live more in my body and in alignment with the actual reality of the life around and within me. The awareness that has arisen from my mindful self-compassion practice has helped me to live according to the truth that I am always unconditionally worthy of my own love. Daily mindful self-compassion not only helps with my physical recovery and ability to cope with chronic pain and chronic self-judgment, but it has played a role in my ability to accept and integrate all parts of my human self.

Part III

Uncovering the True Self
Beneath the Masks

8

There Were Emotional Issues in My Tissues

The Body Is a Book

In paying more attention to my physical body, I discovered that the body is like a book, with repressed emotional events stored within its tissues. Unlike other books, however, the stories within the body cannot be read through thinking but through feeling. With the help of various practitioners who have created safe spaces for me with their own mindful and compassionate attention, I've been able to dive deeper into my body to acknowledge, feel, and integrate the pieces of my life I had previously habitually ignored.

In addition to working with practitioners skilled in Somato-Emotional Release® (SER) and BodyTalk therapy, I also worked with a shiatsu therapist and a naturopath/chiropractor, both of whom had a refined sense of intuition. For instance, the shiatsu therapist only had to raise one of his hands with his palm open toward me for him to sense into the various parts of my body.

"You're working with a male, a patient or a co-worker, who is holding a lot of anger, and you're carrying some of his anger with you," he said during one appointment. He was right.

Earlier that week I had worked with a patient that was angry about his injury, but I was not aware that my body had been holding on to his emotions even after our session had ended.

"You have disappointment in your lungs," he said during another appointment. He was right again, but because I did not yet have a practice of acknowledging uncomfortable emotions, I was not aware of how I was feeling.

As I continued to work with this therapist and the other practitioners mentioned above, I came to learn that I had been carrying emotions from my teenage years, adolescence, and even childhood. I would not have believed the observations these practitioners shared with me if not for the fact that at one point four of them, despite not even knowing each other or being in communication with each other, all made the same observations. After sensing into my body, each one said that something had happened to me at age three or four, an incident in which I had expressed myself honestly but was then reprimanded for speaking my truth. That moment in my childhood was the first time I started to wear masks in order to protect myself.

Though I have not yet been able to recall every part of the specific incident, my dear friend Liezel Annie Palon has been able to help me process the emotions associated with it. Luckily for me, Liezel is a registered massage therapist trained in craniosacral therapy (CST), visceral manipulation, neural manipulation, reiki, and Continuum Movement, as well as SER. One day I went to see Liezel for a body session using SER-via-CST. While lying on the table with Liezel's hands placed on particular parts of my body whose tissues called to be held, all of a sudden I had a vision that felt familiar even though it felt surreal. I saw myself as a three- or four-year-old girl standing in front of dozens of my family and friends. I was holding my very first diary behind my back, hiding it from everyone. I began to feel emotions of sadness for this little girl who felt she had to hide who she was from her own family and friends out of fear of judgment. With Liezel's verbal guidance and her non-judgmental presence, I was able to meet that little girl with acceptance and compassion. There on the table I ended up sobbing. I felt grief not just for the little girl that I had been but also for the adolescent, the teenager, and the adult Jaisa who did not know what it was like to be herself.

Initially I felt anger and grief in coming to acknowledge the truth that I had been repressing my true self at as early as three years old. But in meeting these emotions mindfully, understanding and insight eventually arose and I began to see clearly how my habits in adulthood had been shaped by this childhood incident. Whether it was the mask of "smile and be obedient" or "smile and be happy" or "smile and be grateful," I developed a habit of masking out of the fear of being judged— both by others and myself. Not knowing how to be with emotions that I judged as negative, such as anger and sadness, I coped by layering on mask after mask, not realizing that I was taking away my own right to authentic expression, my own right to be me.

Since that first session with Liezel, I have continued to receive her help to acknowledge more hidden stories within my body. With her skills in SER and CST, I've been able to reacquaint myself with parts of myself I ignored at various ages throughout my life. It appears that the more mindful and compassionate I am when diving in to explore my body, the more I am able to reintegrate and heal. For instance, there was one day in particular when I was able to acknowledge myself at three different stages of my life—when I was twenty-one years old, fourteen years old, and four years old. In just one hour I accessed a part within me where a vision arose of the twenty-one-year-old Jaisa who was at a hip hop party in Toronto, trying so hard to be cool just so that people would like her. I then met the fourteen-year-old Jaisa who was approaching the doors of St. Joseph's College High School on her first day of grade nine. She was scared she would not make any friends and would be alone. But when she walked through the front doors, she saw someone she knew, an acquaintance she had met the year before. Upon hugging her friend, that fourteen-year-old Jaisa felt relief in knowing someone. But it was also in that moment of hugging that the attachment to having many friends, driven by a fear of being alone, began. I then met the five-year-old Jaisa who was with her mom visiting a neighbour who also had a daughter my age. Her daughter, however, was outside playing with the other neighbours. My five-year-old self was looking outside the window feeling angry, sad, and confused as I wondered why I had to stay inside with my mom. With Liezel's guidance I was able to speak to my five-, fourteen-, and twenty-one-year-old self with wisdom, mindfulness, and compassion. In doing so I was finally able to safely feel and express the emotions I had been repressing from those events.

I remained lying on the massage table crying for a few minutes. Liezel allowed me to take my time getting up from the table. When I eventually came to stand up, I noticed that my body felt different. In bringing loving awareness to parts of myself once ignored, I now felt lighter, yet grounded and full.

"This must be what integration feels like," I thought to myself.

Standing up straight and walking around the room felt easier, relative to how I'd felt prior to the session. With my bodily tissues no longer needing to hold onto emotions, my body seemed to have regained potential for more optimal functioning.

"Which tissues do our emotions usually get stuck in?" I later asked Liezel. She replied that emotions can be held anywhere in the body but that sometimes they will be held in our weakest tissues. So when an accident or injury occurs, it is likely that whatever emotions were being experienced during the time of injury, the injured tissue will likely hold those emotions. Because of my own healing journey, I was able to understand Liezel on a palpable level. For instance, I was receiving a medical qigong session one day, when I was guided to explore my body. Going inwards, I felt what I could only describe as "an earthy poo with dark cracks"; it was situated along the length of my spine around the twelfth thoracic vertebra, the exact location of my vertebral fracture and spinal cord compression. Upon mindfully exploring that dark tissue, instantly I went back to a moment in my childhood when my parents were having an argument. With the safe and compassionate guidance of the medical qigong master, I was able to experience the fear I had as that child in that moment.

"I'm afraid my parents will separate," I said.

"What would happen if they did?" the master asked.

"There would be no future possible," I replied. Tears started to roll down my cheeks as I re-experienced the sense of fear I felt in those moments as a child.

The master then guided me to explore with my current wisdom and compassion the possible result if they had separated.

"Life will … life will go on," I realized. At age thirty-seven I had finally come to see that a future would have been possible even if my parents had separated when I was a child.

In bringing that insight to the child that I was, the feeling of fear went away. With the disappearing of that fear arose the realization that this repressed childhood fear of my parents' separating had been subconsciously affecting my behaviours into adulthood. (This is akin to the experience of post-traumatic stress disorder, in which past trauma filters the experience of the present reality.) Because of repressing this fear, I went on to project my expectation that my parents needed to have a perfect marriage. Although my parents' love for each other has grown over the years, I was unable to perceive this reality because the fear stuck in my body was filtering my experience of the present.

It appears that when I broke my back in the motorcycle accident at age thirty, those injured tissues (being the weakest part of my body) absorbed the fears that I still felt around my parents' separation. Now here's an interesting point: my desire to learn how to ride a motorcycle came from my desire to spend more time with my dad, who is a biker, which was also related to the repressed fear of my parents' separating. So when I broke my back, that fear appeared to get stuck in the exact location of the bone fracture and spinal cord compression.

At the end of that medical qigong session I felt lighter and more grounded and was able to move around with more ease. Most interestingly, the pain and tightness in my mid-back decreased. Perhaps it's because I had released a dark, cracked, "earthy poo-like substance" from my tissues.

Not Too Late to Change My Childhood

Prior to my accident and the need for a diversity of therapies, I had no idea that I had an inner child with emotions yet to be acknowledged, wounds yet to be healed. One would think that most of my therapy sessions after the accident would have been about emotions related to the accident and my life with a disability, but in fact most of my sessions revolved around my behaviours that were rooted in childhood.

In discovering that parts of myself were disintegrated, I initially fell into the cow path of blaming my parents, my family, my culture, religion, and society. But it only made me bitter, not better. With mindfulness and compassion I've come to understand that the judgment I give to others is always a reflection of the judgment I give to myself. Accordingly, instead of blaming those who have judged (and inadvertently traumatized) me for simply being honest with my emotions, I can hold others with compassion, acknowledging that the judgment they show me is a reflection of the judgment they hold within themselves.

I consider it one of my greatest feats in life to have compassion for those who have caused me harm. The only way I have been able to significantly extend the boundaries of my compassion is through acknowledging the pains and suffering of the judger, the harmer, and the oppressor.

In 2015, I watched Gabor Maté's play *The Damage Is Done*. There is a scene in which the actor playing the therapist says to the actor playing the patient, "There are no victims or villains, only people in pain." Those words continue to inspire me to see past my own judgments of who is the victim and who is the villain, and to acknowledge that everyone has an inner child who has at least once experienced judgment. With this wisdom, forgiveness and compassion flow more naturally, and while I have not been able to go back in time and change the past, I have been able to change my understanding of my childhood.

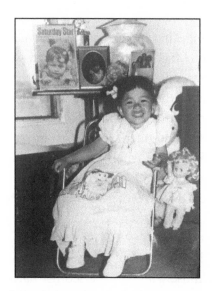

I keep this photo of myself at age
three on my altar to remind myself
to honour my inner child.

More Freedom for Your Life Force to Move through You

While living in Vancouver I met Jane Courtney, a somatic therapist—a body worker—who used to work as a registered nurse in mental health settings. Her background and training in nursing and mental health and her own recovery from traumatic injuries led her to work in body and nervous system health. Wanting to work with upstream solutions and prevention rather than simply treating symptoms, Jane decided to find a practice through which she could address the core of the issues that hold people back in their lives. So, she became a somatic experiencing practitioner and a somatic practice therapist.

Curious to experience her work, I booked three sessions with Jane. What I found interesting over those sessions was how Jane created a particular space where I was encouraged to move freely and notice the sensations and movements of my body; this is the core of somatic experiencing therapy. For instance, instead of feeling obliged to look at her while I sat across from her, I was encouraged to notice what happened when I had the choice to look anywhere I wanted to. I looked to the left, to the right, out the window, around the room; I could look anywhere I wanted to and I found it so simple yet freeing. This process of orienting myself by looking around at the environment helped my body realize it was safe in the present moment.

In each session, Jane would help me explore what I was experiencing in the moment and help my system realize it was safe. With her verbal facilitation, I allowed my body to naturally move in oscillating ways. This was a surprise to me. I had never been aware of my body's natural tendency to oscillate. It turns out we humans are like animals in that after a trauma (big or small) our nervous system processes a single traumatic event experience with a shaking tremor, similarly to how a dog or a cat shakes its body after a traumatic experience. Jane has helped me to understand that she does not work directly with the traumatic event, but rather with the nervous system's response to the event.

"Hold yourself together! Stay composed" is what I often hear from others. Perhaps these common cultural expectations of how I should or should not move have made me judge my body and my need to move in vibrating and oscillating ways. I am reminded of our world's indigenous peoples, who acknowledge this natural movement as medicine and whose traditional dances (many of which mimic the movements of animals) provide safe space for the body to naturally oscillate, vibrate, and shake in healing ways.

After three sessions of experiencing different degrees of bodily shaking, I had a major breakthrough during my last session with Jane. I started to experience a sensation that felt like a piece of wood was blocking the top of my throat. Jane asked, "I'm curious. Was a neck collar ever placed on you during your accident?"

"Yes, after I got injured, the paramedics put a collar on me before they put me on the plinth," I replied. As soon as I recalled the moment when the collar was placed on my neck, something inside me was triggered.

Then the thought arose: "I can't move my legs!"

As feelings of fear arose I began to cry and wail out loud. I continued crying for another five or so minutes. The release felt good. However, I was confused because I had not experienced any fear either in the moments after the accident or in the ambulance.

"Where is all this emotion coming from? I didn't experience any fear when I broke my back," I asked Jane. She replied by saying what many others have told me. Apparently, in the hours after my accident, I didn't experience any fear because I was in shock.

I emailed Jane the next day, saying, "Hi, Jane. After our sessions, would you believe that two different people I met up with thought I looked either amazing or like I just went on a relaxing vacation? I'm also feeling like I have more creativity in the last few days."

Jane explained how I was showing signs of greater nervous system regulation. Since I was no longer unconsciously managing my nervous system activation (from the shock that locked me in freeze mode), my creativity now had more space.

In Jane's words, "Our bodies have a record of everything that has happened to us, and the unprocessed traumas can leave us living a life that is less full than it could be. Once the trauma has been processed, there is more room and more freedom for life force to emerge and move through you. This results in greater capacity and resilience and greater nervous system regulation."

This life force that Jane spoke of is energy—life force energy. It flows through the body and is charged by strong emotional experiences. Through my explorations with somato-emotional release I've come to appreciate the word "emotion" as "e-motion" where "e" stands for energy; thus e-motion is energy-in-motion.

Feelings are meant to be fleeting. Emotions are meant to move. But when emotions are repressed due to judgment and/or trauma, the natural movement of life force energy flowing through the body becomes stagnant. There is no motion for the e-motion.

So herein again comes the role of compassion and mindfulness, which hones my ability to be in community with all of our humanity's emotions, with curiosity, patience, non-judgment, and acceptance. In the practice of medical qigong, the body is actually acknowledged for its ability to process the continuum of human emotions. For instance, the lungs are the energetic container for both grief and integrity; the kidneys contain both fear and inner wisdom; the liver holds anger and compassion; the heart processes overexcitement, peace, order, and harmony; and the spleen processes both worry and trust. Through these Eastern lenses I am inspired to allow any emotion to be part of the present moment. In doing so, I can integrate all the different aspects of myself to be parts of the whole that I am.

9

Waking Up to the Energy Body

Dare Not Say "Energy"

"New age hippy dippy woo-woo." That's how I used to refer to people who did any type of energy work such as reiki.

I judged those who provided energy work, assuming they did not have a sufficiently academic background and thus their work was less worthy of respect than the Western medicine I studied myself. In truth, I was jealous of energy healers because I thought it was not fair that I had spent so much time and money on three university degrees in order to be a scientific-evidence-based therapist and I assumed that all energy healers had not.

Mostly, I judged energy work because I myself was not aware of the life force energy flowing through my body. I did not learn about the concept of an energy body in elementary school, high school, or even post-secondary school. Despite having a bachelor's degree both in education and in physical and health education (PHE) and a two-year master's degree in occupational therapy (OT), I had only once heard the energy body being acknowledged. This once was during a tai chi class that was offered as one of the practicum choices for students of the PHE program. Interestingly, that program has since been changed, with the number of practicums being decreased. I find this unfortunate because practicums are what provide us with embodied experiences of physical activity, strengthening our sense of intuition and body-knowing, and balancing out the intellectual head-knowing. Who knows, if it were not for that one tai chi practicum, the seed of energy awareness might not have been planted in my own anti-energy mindset.

The Problem with Cadavers

As part of the PHE and OT programs that I completed, I enjoyed numerous opportunities to learn more about the human body through working with cadavers. I enjoyed learning about the human body so much that I ended up excelling in anatomy, and so after graduation I went on to become an anatomy lab instructor for ten years as part of the OT department's status-only program. From 2005 to 2015, I helped OT students navigate the human cadaver—its bones, muscles, tendons, and ligaments—and facilitated their understanding of how our human structure affects our daily functions. Unfortunately, my move to Vancouver in 2015 meant that I had to let go of this instructor position. However, in stepping away from the experience I gained a broader perspective.

My Western academic mind's understanding of health and wellness was limited to what I learned from working with dead tissue, where the vital essence animating life is missing. In a cadaver, we will not find the breath. In a cadaver, we will not find the flow of fluids. In a cadaver, we will not find life force energy, or as practitioners of traditional Chinese medicine (TCM) call it "chi," as in "tai chi" (also spelled "qi" in qigong and "ki" in reiki).

Unlike Western medicine, Eastern medical systems, including TCM and the Indian Vedic system (which includes

Ayurvedic medicine and yoga), acknowledge and are aware of the energy that flows through the body and how integral it is to health and healing. It is from these Eastern systems of knowledge that I am learning about the anatomy of the energy body and the various ways it can be described. For instance, I am now aware that we have energy centres within our body, the largest of which are along our spinal column from the sacrum to the skull. Some systems of knowledge refer to these energy centres as chakras and others refer to them as dantians. I find it interesting as a neuro-rehab OT with a spinal cord injury how these energy centres follow the path of the central nervous system—the brain and the spinal cord—which are full of neurons that light up with electrical impulses. What I find intriguing about the energy body is that it exists not just within the physical body but beyond it, with its energy field extending far beyond the skin. I've heard many refer to our energy field as an aura, and in TCM it is referred to as the wei qi field.

Using Our Natural Senses

While it's still highly beneficial to learn physical anatomy from dead tissue, we can enhance our understanding of the living body by paying mindful attention to our own living body and the life force energy that runs through it.

I used to think that only those who were gifted with extra senses could sense life force energy. But in spending more time with my friend Sharon Brant, who is visually impaired, I started to discover that almost every human being has the potential to sense the flow (or lack of flow) of energy through the body's natural sense perceptions.

Despite losing her vision at age nine, Sharon continues to live life to the fullest. She commutes to her full-time job in downtown Toronto; volunteers as a Rick Hansen Foundation Ambassador, speaking to youth about living with a disability; and is a wife, a mother of two, and a good friend to many, including me. After my accident, Sharon and I would plan regular trips to the spa together, after which we would normally walk somewhere to grab a bite. One day we returned to a restaurant that had gone through renovations since our last visit. While waiting for our meals to arrive, Sharon commented on how much larger the windows were and how much higher the ceilings seemed. I was surprised because I myself, with twenty/twenty vision, was unaware of the renovations she'd observed.

"How can you tell?" I asked.

"I can sense it," she replied. She went on to describe how she can tell when a room in her home is clean versus cluttered. This boggled my mind because Sharon is not an intuitive, nor someone who has extra senses. But with the loss of her vision, over time she has cultivated her other natural human senses, allowing her to better perceive her surroundings.

Sharon's ability to develop her senses made me curious to explore how much more of life I could perceive if I cultivated my natural human senses. I figured that if I was not even noticing things with my eyes that a person with a visual impairment could sense, then perhaps I could sense life force energy if I just learned to pay more attention through my natural senses.

One person who helped me to sense the energy in my body is chiropractor Allison Barriscale, DC, a provider of Network Spinal Analysis (NSA) and Somato Respiratory Integration (SRI). When I first started to work with Dr. Barriscale in 2014, she would have me lie down on the chiropractic table and focus on the sensations of breath, movement, and energy. I had no problems observing the sensations of breath and the movements in my body caused by breathing, but when it came to observing energy I was confused. I had never paid specific attention to energy in my body, so I did not know what I was supposed to be looking for. Dr. Barriscale explained to me that different people perceive energy differently. For instance, some may experience energy in the body as light or even particular colours, while others may experience the energy as heat, coolness, buzzing, or a sense of stagnancy. Because I had never paid attention to the energy body before the accident, I had a misconception that perceiving energy would be a surreal, mystical experience. Turns out, perceiving life force energy can be as simple as feeling tingling in my arms or a density in the air like a misty cloud around my skin. Whether it's energy within our bodies or energy in the environment, such as tension, love in the air, or feel-bad and feel-good vibes, we can perceive frequencies of energy with our natural human senses.

Since waking up to the reality of the energy body, I have expanded my mindfulness practice to include not just the tissues of my physical body but also the energy centres and meridians along which life force energy flows within my body. With the fresh new eyes of beginner's mind, I am enjoying the daily discovery of how it feels to have life force energy flowing through me. Now, if someone like me who used to hardly feel my own feet on the ground can cultivate the ability to sense the energy body, then I believe everyone else has the potential to do so too.

From Newtonian to Quantum Understanding

I love science and the humility that inherently comes in applying the scientific method to learning about life. For instance, how humbling it is that every single good research study always ends with something along the lines of "but further research needs to be done." Unfortunately though, Western medicine has been limited to the box of the Newtonian sciences, in which an object must be perceived through the five human senses so it can be measured, experimented with, and predicted. For instance, the Newtonian mindset will confirm that I have a physical body because we can easily see and measure the mass of the physical body, and thus we can predict that it will succumb to the forces of gravity. The energy body, on the other hand, does not obey the laws of Newtonian physics, simply because the particles that make up the energy body are so miniscule in mass that that they have no gravitational pull. In other words, the energy body is so minute in density and weight that it does not follow the Newtonian understanding of how matter and gravity function. Thus, the energy body cannot be understood from a Newtonian mindset.

To understand the energy body better, I had to learn to start thinking outside the box of the Newtonian mindset and integrate the science of quantum physics. The world of quantum science explores our nature at the smallest scale of existence, such as at the level of atoms and subatomic particles. It is with this more in-depth way of exploring our existence that I have been better able to understand life force energy and how it relates to healing.

It is also important to acknowledge the colonial roots of Western medicine, for it has played a role in limiting the expansion of the medical sciences beyond Newtonian ways of thinking. Colonization has a long history of marginalizing not just indigenous peoples but their different knowledge and systems of healing and medicine. The traditional medicine of indigenous peoples has always been holistic, acknowledging not just the physical aspects of being human but the mental, emotional, energetic, and spiritual aspects as well, while Western medicine has only just begun to acknowledge the mental and emotional aspects of human health, and it has yet to integrate the role of energy and spirit. It is through using this limited way of understanding the human body that some practitioners of Western medicine have come to judge the notion of the energy body. Just as that doctor from Sunnybrook broke me down, making me feel like a fool for believing in energy-based modalities, resistance toward acknowledging the energy body can cause people harm. That being said, I must admit that I myself have not only been the one harmed but have been the one to cause harm to others through my own Newtonian ways of thinking.

I Judged My Patient

In 2005, my first year of working as an OT, I had a patient admitted to an inpatient medical rehab unit. She had a diagnosis of fibromyalgia and chronic fatigue, with symptoms so severe that she needed help with all her daily personal care. We initially had a good relationship based on trust and respect, but things changed when she brought her reiki healer to provide sessions inside her room.

I recall reacting with judgment when my patient told me about her reiki practice. I judged not only the practice of reiki as being "hippy dippy nonsense" that had no scientific basis, but in turn I also judged my patient for believing this nonsense would help her. Interestingly, everyone else on this patient's multi-disciplinary healthcare team also judged reiki as being weird and of no benefit to our patient. The act of receiving reiki, on top of the fact that the patient's symptoms were labelled by the team as "psychosomatic" (meaning caused by mental factors), cast a negative light on the patient. Consequently, the patient's symptoms were not taken seriously, and we decided as a team to discharge her despite her saying she wanted to stay longer to receive more therapy.

Out of the hundreds of patients I've worked with over the years, this patient has stayed on my mind. "How did she do after discharge? How is she today?" I've asked myself. The answers to these questions I don't know, and for a long time I held on to feelings of guilt around how I judged her. I have been able to move forward, however, using this experience as an opportunity to practice humility, self-forgiveness, and mindfulness toward energy-based modalities and the people who practise them.

Game-Changing Exercises

With a curiosity to understand the energy body, I went on to complete my first- and second-degree certifications in the Usui system of reiki, an introduction to Emotional Freedom Technique, and several workshops of the Healing from the Core series with Suzanne Scurlock-Durana, including "Advanced Energy Dynamics" and "Full Body Presence, Grounding, and Healthy Boundaries." Currently, I am in the Medical Qigong and Chinese Shamanic Medicine programs at the Empty Mountain Institute, where I completed the practitioner certifications in 2017 and will eventually become a therapist in 2019 and a master by 2021.

Throughout these courses I've had the opportunity to engage in various exercises that have expanded my mind to new ways of experiencing the energy body.

More Awareness Equals More Power

One exercise that blew my mind open was an exploration in raising my physical, energetic, and spiritual arm. On the first attempt I was to lift my arm with awareness of only my physical arm, and on the second attempt I was to lift my arm with an expanded awareness that included my energetic arm. On the third attempt I was to lift my arm with an even more expanded awareness that included my spiritual arm.

"Holy shit," I thought to myself, feeling surprised. Raising my arm with awareness of both the physical and the energetic arm actually made lifting my arm easier. But lifting my arm with all three levels of the body—the physical, energetic, and spiritual—made lifting my arm the easiest.

Ever since that exercise, I've continued to explore, expanding my awareness beyond my physical body to include the energetic and spiritual bodies when doing physically taxing activities. For instance, when I am outside carrying heavy groceries and I feel myself getting tired, if for some reason I cannot stop to rest, I experiment connecting with my energetic and spiritual bodies. Every time I do this, I experience a second wind, as if I've tapped into a backup engine that allows me to keep moving with less pain and more stamina.

Energy Follows Attention

Also, a series of exercises has shown me that I can actually direct the flow of energy with my own cultivated attention. My first experience of this concept was when I learned how to fill my body up with life force energy through my feet. All I had to do was pay attention to my body and the ground beneath me, and visualize roots connecting me to the earth and its life force energy. At first I judged myself as a weirdo for even attempting this, but when I looked around to see if my fellow classmates were doing it, not only did I see them all doing it, but I realized that many of them were healthcare professionals like myself. If they were open to this exercise, then maybe it wasn't as woo-woo as I thought. So on with the exercise I went, and as I paid attention to my feet—visualizing the earth's energy entering through the bottoms of my feet, going up my legs, and filling up the rest of my body—the energy actually flowed.

"Maybe I'm just imagining this," I thought. But I eventually learned that imagination should not be discredited as something unreal, for it is the skill of imagining that allows us to cultivate the energy body.

When I first started to consciously receive life force energy from the earth, I couldn't feel it myself, but my teachers and several of my classmates could sense it and would even tell me when my body was full enough with energy.

"Okay, stop. You're juicy enough!" my teacher Suzanne Scurlock-Durana would often say.

But with repeated practice over the years and the wonder of neuroplasticity, I have been able to develop my sense perceptions and can now feel life force energy moving up my legs and filling my body like a very mild but palpable moist cloud. With the cultivation of my mind through a regular meditation practice, I am also better able to direct my attention, and accordingly I'm better able to direct the flow of life force energy both within and around my body.

Another exercise demonstrating how energy really does follow attention is when my classmates and I were to pair up and sense into each other's energy body. When my partner first sensed into my energy body, she noticed that most of my energy was situated above my waist. That made sense to me because, with paralysis being from the waist down, I paid less attention to my legs and feet. Furthermore, as I am an overthinker, most of my energy would consequently be up in my head. After I did a short body scan, paying more attention to my feet and legs, my partner sensed back into my body and she could tell that my energy body was more grounded in my legs and feet.

"Wow, so all I have to do is pay more attention to my legs and feet, and the energy will follow," I thought.

Curious to explore the correlation between life force energy and neural rewiring, I became motivated to bring more attention and energy to my lower extremities in the hopes it would improve my functional recovery.

Everything Is Energy

The final exercise I'll share is one that opened my mind to the notion that everything in this universe, including the body, is energy. This exercise involves a table with a white tablecloth on top of which are circles cut out of fabric of various colours. With each piece of fabric cut into the same size, the only difference between the circles was their colour. My classmates and I were to walk around this table and place our hands above each circle, palpating the vibrations each different colour gave off.

"No way," I initially thought.

Until I did this exercise, I had never experienced feeling the different vibrations that different colours give off. As I walked around with my open palms a few centimetres above each coloured fabric, I felt nothing; I only felt jealousy of the rest of my classmates who claimed they could feel the difference between the colours. I was discouraged up until I palpated the energy of one circle that had rainbow stripes. As I waved my hands from side to side over this rainbow-striped fabric, I felt as if I was running my palms over corduroy. I was so shocked, I actually had to take a closer look at the fabric to make sure it was in fact a flat piece of fabric and not corduroy. But upon inspection, the fabric was clearly flat and the corduroy sensation I palpated with my palms was from the differing vibrations of the rainbow-coloured stripes.

While my mind has always known that different colours are just different frequencies of the energy of light, I never knew it from a bodily sense of knowing. I went away from that exercise thinking, "Wow, so everything is energy!"

10

From Repression to Creative Expression

Healing with Words

With a broader perception of everything around me being different forms and frequencies of energy, I began to understand how the various arts, including the movement arts and the musical, visual, dramatic, and lyrical arts, are different ways of bringing motion to emotions. My curiosity led me to explore how creative expression through different art mediums would provide healing emotional release. I took classes in weaving, Chinese brush painting, therapeutic writing, improv, and stand-up comedy. But the most consistent medium of creative expression for me has been the use of both the written and the spoken word. With few people to take my masks off to, I began journaling young. Writing in a diary was one of the few safe spaces for my honest expression, so I knew for a long time that writing is a cathartic practice.

The Written Word

A year after the accident I created a blog called *Memoirs of a Jaisa* as a platform to express myself at different points along my healing journey. I shared journal excerpts, reflections, and even poetry.

Pre-injury, I rarely wrote poems, but post-injury I found poetry to be an avenue for me to express emotions that I was not in the habit of acknowledging. For instance, in December 2013 I was in a session with my BodyTalk practitioner Linda Eales. It was a session I'll never forget, because that was the day that I first welcomed anger. I grew up thinking that anger was a "bad" and "negative" emotion, so if ever I did feel angry, I would follow the emotional experience usually with emotions of guilt and thoughts of "I feel bad" just for having felt angry. Linda explained to me that anger can be a catalyst for change and thus a wonderfully powerful energy.

After my session with Linda that day, I went to a nearby café to grab a coffee. The combination of Linda's BodyTalk session and her pep talk on anger had mobilized something inside me. While sitting at a table sipping a cup of coffee, I felt something arising from within my body. I felt the urge to pull my laptop out of my bag and open up a new Word document. I looked at the blank page on my computer screen for a few moments when all of a sudden I felt a sensation in my throat. It was a new feeling to me. I placed both hands on the keyboard and next thing I knew, I found myself typing the letters "A, N, G, E, R." As soon as I saw the word, tears welled up in my eyes and my fingers started to type incredibly quickly, as if a faucet had opened at the tips of my fingers. The following words just flowed out:

ANGER

Eyes tearing
Samba playing
Horns
Cowbells
Warmth in my eyes

This bar ... called Lit Espresso
How appropriate
For something in me has been lit
An anger
Why me?
Tears
Flowing
I'm holding it in
My eyeliner must not come off.

Movers and shakers
Movers and shakers
My teacher says anger is great!
It can move you
It can shift you

Tears
The smell of coffee beans
Roasted
Dark
Chatter
People
Perhaps they too chatter of the pain they have
The anger they have

Ahh ...
I feel it in my throat
A burning
A yearning
To cry and tell the world
Poor me!
Poor me!
Dammit
My eyeliner is ruined.

Just grateful I'm alive
Just grateful I'm alive
Ah yes, how gratitude got me through things
But wait.
What's this inside me?
In my heart, there is anger?
In my heart, there are tears?
I did not know my heart has been yearning to be heard
Felt
Held

Held
It's all running
My eyes. My nose
Running

And the samba plays on
The lineup for espressos continues on
A stranger asks: "Are you okay?"
"Oh yes. I'm just writing some poetry that is taking me
somewhere."

Somewhere
Somewhere
Deep
To a place I have not explored
Until now

Ahh
A warmth in my back
A loosening in my throat
Eyes numb from this paper towel napkin

But Deeper my breath goes
Deeper I inhale
Deeper I exhale
Deeper I drop
Into this moment

The horns
The cowbells
The chatter
The people

All go on
As does this anger
As does this pain
As do I
As do I

This child beside me
Waiting for her hot chocolate
Wonders
Why?
Why the tears?

Anger I say
Pain I feel

But I am fine, child.
I am fine.

For all goes on
And I go on
I
GO
ON

I wrote this poem in one go. No thinking. Just feeling and typing. I was amazed. I could not believe that I had repressed these emotions of anger about my accident for almost three and a half years. I felt like I had just met my shadow, a dark part of myself that had been following me but that I had never acknowledged until that afternoon. Meeting and integrating this exiled part of myself left me feeling more whole. Feeling indeed was proving to be healing.

Half a year after writing "Anger," I was with my social worker Tracy Martin, who recommended that I explore writing to express my grief around loss related to the accident. In particular she recommended that I write a eulogy, because it had been almost four years after my injury and I had not yet expressed any grief. I had been so focused on just feeling grateful for being alive with no head injury and having a supportive community that I thought I should have no reason to grieve. The layered masks of "smile and be grateful" had distanced me from the part of myself deep inside that felt sadness over the loss of being able to walk barefoot. But with a four-year-long relationship of trust with Tracy, I decided to take her word for it and put my words into the following eulogy to barefoot walking:

A Eulogy to Barefoot Walking 1980–2010

Family and friends, colleagues and strangers, thank you for taking the time to remember Barefoot Walking with me (a.k.a. B.W. or B-Dub for short).

B-Dub came into my world just before I turned one (supposedly beating the rest of my friends at my age). By the time I started kindergarten, B-Dub had already begun exploring the art of ballet and Hawaiian dancing. With the support of my mom, I was later able to participate in competitions across North America, dancing jazz, tap, lyrical ballet, and Hawaiian.

When I turned eighteen, however, B-Dub felt the need to ground itself in older roots. So, I decided to join Folklorico Filipino Canada (FFC), a folk dance group that I ended up dancing with until the summer of 2010, when an accident happened. B-Dub allowed me to do so much over those twelve years with FFC, such as perform at weddings and festivals and, my favourite, tour across the world!

Considering the majority of Filipino folk dances are performed barefoot, the amazing B-Dub allowed me to be one of the group's Muslim vinta princesses, which required that I dance while balancing on top of two bamboo sticks atop two men's shoulders. I was also one of the group's tinikling dancers, jumping between bamboo sticks that close together on every beat. This dance—tinikling—is the Philippine national dance, which depicts the tikling birds hopping between bamboo sticks; it was one of my favourites.

B-Dub, however, was not always in the spotlight for its skills. Many made fun of B-Dub, calling it "veiny," "skinny," and, the most common, "hammer toes." When I was at St. Mary's Elementary School, I took part in an after-school program where I received the "Ugliest Feet Award." B-Dub knew, though, that its beauty lay in its function. I will never forget how ballet teachers would envy B-Dub for the "beautiful point" it was able to reach with its high arch.

If B-Dub didn't know it was loved and appreciated then, I know it does now.

While it's been almost four years since B-dub was last here, I have the utmost faith in its resurrection. I do believe it will return again. I may not know when, but I know that when it does, I will not be taking it for granted.

Just like during the writing of the poem "Anger," my tears flowed as I wrote this eulogy, because it made me acknowledge all of the meaningful activities that barefoot walking had allowed me to do. In losing "B-Dub," I lost everything that it allowed. I shared the eulogy with my social worker, close friends, and family. It felt good to have my grief met with acceptance, not just by myself but by my community as well.

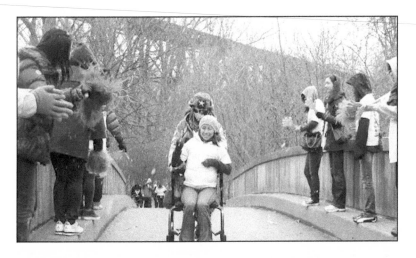

My father and I crossing the finish line of the 2013 5k Walk for Multiple Sclerosis. Due to pain and fatigue I was unable to walk the whole 5k so my parents and friends took turns pushing me while I sat on my rollater walker. At that time I was not aware that my smile was masking anger and sadness due to feeling limited and dependent on others.

The Spoken Word

At the end of one of my mindfulness trainings in 2012, the teachers held a talent night where course participants were invited to share music, song, and poetry. I decided to recite a poem that I had written called "That Thing." It was received well and I was encouraged by many to look into speaking at poetry slams. So upon returning home from that course, together with my friend Monique Lyn (who was willing to share her poetry as well), I mustered up enough courage to go to Dwayne Morgan's Roots Lounge Open Mic and Poetry Slam at Toronto's Harlem Restaurant. I got a few finger snaps that night, enough encouragement to keep me motivated, to keep me expressing myself through spoken word. With the freedom to choose my tone, volume, pace, and rhythm, the spoken word grants me many ways to creatively bring motion to the emotions I describe with each word.

For the first few years after starting my *Memoirs of a Jaisa* blog, I posted many poems, unaware that one day a stranger would be moved by my words. Linda Spencer was that stranger, who eventually became a friend. She encouraged me to submit my poems to a contest by Sibella, an online poetry magazine that publishes women's poetry from around the world. Not only did I win that contest, where the prize included having my poetry published in every bimonthly issue for one year, but I also won the opportunity to fly to San Miguel de Allende in Mexico to be a keynote speaker and a workshop facilitator for their Women's Spirituality and Wellness Expo.

I decided to share a reflection on my healing journey in a talk called "The Love Journey: Moving from a Place Without to a Place Within." Being able to share my story in my own creative way and have it be witnessed with love and acceptance by so many at that expo made me feel like I was a weak flame that had been fueled into a bonfire. Also, the opportunity to offer a workshop of my own creation at the expo in Mexico challenged me to put myself out there for people to receive. And while only two people signed up for my three-hour workshop called "Self-Compassion: From Creating Our Own Suffering to Giving Our Love," the exchange that transpired between me and those two participants was so rich that I am still friends with them today. That trip to Mexico showed me that various ways of sharing my words heal me and others. Since then I've gone on to do more talks and facilitate workshops as creative ways of not just expressing myself but to help others heal too.

Expressive Arts Therapy

I am fortunate to have a friend in Toronto named Andrea Mapili who is a Tamalpa practitioner, which means that she is certified in the professional application of the Tamalpa Life/Art Process, an approach that integrates imagination, movement, and dance to connect us to the wisdom of the body. Andrea also specializes in movement-based expressive arts therapy and education. If not for her, it might have taken me much longer to discover the healing work of expressive arts therapy. I've come to learn that expressive arts therapy is different from traditional art expression in that it concentrates on the process rather than on the end product. For instance, to honour the idea that my life is a tapestry of emotional experiences, I started a project involving weaving in which the yarn colour and changing patterns I chose represented emotions of grief and anger from my accident. When I was halfway into the project, I had released enough emotions in the process that I didn't even bother to finish what I'd started.

I've had several sessions with Andrea, and what surprises me about her work is the lesson that we can access emotions in the body through the simple act of moving the body. For instance, our sessions would begin with Andrea playing music and creating a safe space for me to move my body freely without any sense of judgment. She would lead me in a guided movement exploration, allowing me to move as my body wanted. After this movement portion, she would give me paper and coloured oil pastels and guide me to draw in response to the movement, using whatever shapes and lines I felt called to draw. After that I would then be given a pen to write words. With every session I would be surprised at the words I wrote that reflected emotions I was not aware I was holding inside my body. What I love most about Andrea's work is that all of the words, colours, and shapes that unfolded began with me accessing them through the movement of the body. Living outside my body for so long, I was surprised at how much information could come through in just the simple act of moving my body.

"How does that work?" I asked Andrea.

She responded by reminding me that before there were words, the body was the medium for language.

"This notion that the body is the medium for language coincides well with the other notion that the body is a book," I thought.

Touring internationally with Folklorico Filipino Canada and seeing many countries' traditional dances has taught me that the most universal way to express the stories of the body is to move it. So with a deeper appreciation for the expression that comes with moving, I sought to incorporate dancing into my rehabilitation.

Healing through Dance

I have to thank my good friend Blessyl Buan, DC, a chiropractor, Pilates instructor, and dance artist, for being the first practitioner to tell me "Jaisa, you will dance again."

In addition to our traditional chiropractic treatments, Dr. Blessyl introduced and coached modified dance movements in the dance studio that transformed into my healing space. Dr. Blessyl and I worked collaboratively with Darryl Tracy, who is not only one of my physiotherapists but also a dance artist and senior faculty member at the School of Toronto Dance Theatre. Together, Dr. Blessyl and Darryl helped me to explore dancing in new ways that were safe for my body. Initially, we explored creative movements lying and sitting on the floor.

Later we moved on to exploring expressive movement from a seated position on a chair or a barstool.

With every session I felt an array of emotions coming through my movements. I can still recall feeling despair while on my hands and knees with my head hanging low, rocking side to side. Another time I felt so frustrated as I squeezed my fists tightly and rocked my head up and down, as if I was trying to get my thoughts out of my head. When I felt free to creatively move my body, my face seemed to join in with the movement as well. Noticing the sensations in my face while I dance, I was surprised at how much sadness and anger was reflected through the squinching of my face, the dropping of my jaw, and the furrowing of my eyebrows and forehead. Until then, I thought dance was usually a joyful act. I appreciated the realization that I can dance with whatever emotion I feel.

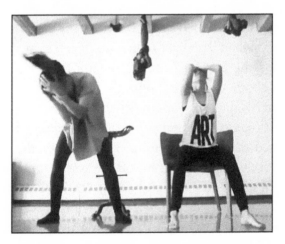

With Dr. Blessyl Buan (standing to my right) exploring new ways to dance from a seated position.

With the creative expression, bodily engagement, and emotional release that occurred in each of my dance sessions with Dr. Blessyl and Darryl, I always observed an improvement in my posture and gait. But perhaps even more important was my renewed confidence in my ability to dance. My last session with Dr. Blessyl occurred just before my move to Vancouver, and we actually ended with a dance battle. We didn't care who won. We were both just happy that I was able to express myself confidently through more ways of moving my body.

I eventually became a member of Ecstatic Dance Toronto, a non-profit that provides a safe space for individuals to dance freely within a community setting. Upon my first time experiencing ecstatic dancing, I was humbled in the discovery that I had been dancing in my head for most of my life. As a child who took jazz, tap, ballet, lyrical, and Hawaiian dance lessons, I performed routines according to choreography that I had to memorize, so I was actually in my head more than in my body when I danced. Performing in competitions in Canada and the US, I had to make sure that I remembered the taught choreography, in hopes that my dance group would impress the competition judges. With ecstatic dance, however, no one is watching or judging. Instead, the ecstatic dance space is considered sacred, with reminders to honour the body and move how one wishes. The music always starts slowly, then builds to an energetic peak and ends with meditative sounds. Speaking to each other is not allowed on the ecstatic dance floor, which allows the dancer to focus inward. In the few times I've gone, I felt not only more connected to my body but more connected to the people around me.

Our Ancestors Danced

At age thirty-six, I was horrified to learn that, upon colonization, many of the Philippines' indigenous healers and shamans (referred to by the Visayan term "babaylan") were killed and fed to crocodiles. Over three hundred years of colonization caused generations in my lineage to forget their ancestral medicine, so that my own parents were not aware the babaylan even existed until I told them. In honour of my ancestors, I have begun to explore the ways in which they healed. In addition to learning about Philippine herbs and medicinal foods, I'm learning that this gathering together of a community to dance to rhythms and music was a part of their traditional medicine.

When I moved to Vancouver I joined the Kathara Pilipino Indigenous Arts Collective Society. In 2003 its co-founders, Babette Santos and Elenita Boots Dumlao, were adopted by the Bagobo Tagabawa Tribe via immersion and cultural exchange, and have since been given permission by the tribe to share their indigenous music, songs, and dances. I joined Kathara in 2016, the same year they started their collaboration with Butterflies in Spirit, a Vancouver-based dance group started by Lorelei Williams, whose mission is to raise awareness around missing and murdered indigenous women and girls across Canada.

Witnessing the collaboration between Kathara and Butterflies in Spirit has taught me that engaging in music, song, and dance is a common way that many of our Filipino and First Nations ancestors healed, and an ongoing way of healing. What I found beautiful about the work between Kathara and Butterflies in Spirit was the exchange of each culture's medicine through the sharing and integrating of each other's music, song, and dance into one collaborative piece. Whenever we got together to make music, sing, and dance, we honoured our shared pains, both present and intergenerational, and we always left our practices and performances feeling physically, emotionally, and spiritually better.

I used to think that only a physician could be the provider of medicine. So it has been very humbling for me as a Western-trained healthcare professional to open my eyes to the fact that dancing, singing, and making music together in community can be medicine.

11

If the Soul Can Leave, It Can Return

Soul Retrieval

In 2012 I was at the Omega Institute in Rhinebeck, New York, for a weeklong mindfulness course with Jon Kabat-Zinn. The course schedule allowed for some free time, so I decided to use my free time by signing up for one of the services at the Omega Wellness Center. Scanning the list of services offered, I was surprised to see shamanic healing. I had never been to a space that offered shamanic services before, so I was quick to jump on this opportunity.

To my surprise, the shaman was not what I expected. I thought I would be meeting with an old indigenous-looking elder. Instead, the shaman who worked with me was an American-born blonde Caucasian woman who had studied shamanic work in the United States.

"You're a shaman?" I thought in my head, doubting her abilities.

Inside her office were paintings and photographs of various animals. The shaman gave me some time to look around. After some dialogue, she had me lie back in a foldout lawn chair with my eyes closed while she went on to drum and embark on what she said would be a journey. I was tempted to open my eyes and sneak a peek at what she was doing, but I was afraid I'd get in trouble, so I kept my eyes shut. At one point she stopped drumming and told me that she'd met a part of my soul that was a toddler. She saw my toddler soul in a backyard sitting at a table, creating arts and crafts and having fun with other children. The shaman then told me that my toddler soul had had to leave my physical body around age three or four, at a specific moment when she didn't feel safe.

"Would you like to welcome your soul back?" the shaman asked me.

"Yes," I responded, even though I did not know how that was going to happen.

The shaman then continued to drum again, and from what I could hear, it sounded as though she was making movements around my body. She then moved toward the top of my head and blew air into the crown of my head. I later came to understand that this was the moment she helped my toddler soul reinhabit my body.

I walked out of her office feeling confused. That was my first experience with the practice of soul retrieval. It was not until two years later, when I had the various practitioners telling me that I had started to wear masks when I was reprimanded for expressing myself at age three or four, that I put two and two together. I started to open up to the possibility that in being judged for expressing my true self, my soul felt unsafe to reside within me and therefore left my physical body.

Mask Meditations

Curiosity has led me to find other ways of retrieving parts of my disintegrated soul. As part of my certification to become a practitioner of medical qigong, I've had to listen to numerous meditations guided by my teacher Wendy Lang. One of these meditations is called a mask meditation, and it can be considered another form of soul retrieval.

I do this meditation regularly now, so I can share one of my experiences to demonstrate how it helps me. In the beginning of the meditation, I am guided to acknowledge the layers of masks that I have been wearing as coping and defence mechanisms. Every time I do this meditation, I am to work with just one of the layers of masks. The most common mask that has been layered on thick is my "smile, I am happy" mask. After acknowledging this mask, I am then guided to take the mask off, noticing how it feels when it's off and then noticing how it feels when I put it back on. The meditation guides me to explore my relationship with this mask with questions such as "How has this mask served me and how does it no longer serve me?"

Within the safe container that mindfulness and compassion create, I have been able to discover how the "smile, I am happy" mask has defended me from the risk of having my true emotions judged when expressed. Some human emotions are naturally unpleasant to feel, so if I express them outwardly I risk being judged by those who cannot sit with the discomfort themselves. Now, this mask has not only defended me but it has served as a coping mechanism by allowing me to please those with unconscious expectations that I be happy. If others are not feeling good, my "smile, I am happy" mask often makes them feel better. So from this stance of understanding, I have been able to appreciate how this mask was of good service to others and myself in the past.

In the present, however, this mask no longer serves me, because with it on I feel a sense of imprisonment, of not allowing myself to be myself. During these mask meditations, whenever I take off this "smile, I am happy" mask, I feel free to feel whatever I feel, even if it's not deemed positive by others. With the mask off, I can feel angry, confused, doubtful, apprehensive, and scared, yet in having it off I can also feel excited, happy, and motivated. In tasting the freedom that comes with feeling all my emotions, I get a taste of what it's like to be fully alive.

The next part of the meditation requires beginner's mind, non-judgment, and trust. After acknowledging how the mask no longer serves a purpose, I then go on to ask the mysterious divine to transform the energy of this mask into pure light. Once the mask is transformed I ask the divine to return this pure light to me. This reclaiming of divine light as part of who I am is akin to the retrieval of a part of my soul.

A Safe Space for the Soul to Be

Through my training in medical qigong I'm learning that there are three worlds, and so accordingly we also have three bodies: the physical, the energetic, and the spiritual. The energy world lies between the physical and the spiritual, connecting the two worlds. As such, energy is required for spirit to manifest in the physical form of the human body. The extent to which life force energy flows through my body determines how much of my soul I can embody. Hence why yoga can be healing, because it promotes the flow of this vital life force energy (also called "prana" in Sanskrit), thus also deepening our connection to spirit.

Perhaps it is a good thing that the soul has the ability to leave the physical body as a way to defend itself from the judgments and trauma that seem to come with human living. However, I know that my soul has not come here to this physical world just so that it can check out of my body for most of my life. I know my soul came here for a reason.

To Evolve and Express My Love

With spirit and soul being unquantifiable by science, it is not common for practitioners of Western healthcare to speak of these terms with their patients. Yet the few times that a healthcare practitioner has explicitly referred to my soul have felt like the quenching of a thirst I never knew I had.

For instance, while in Vancouver I continued to receive regular Network Spinal Analysis (NSA) from Joyce Chen, DC. After most NSA entrainments, I feel waves of energy flowing up and down my spine, from my sacrum to my cranium. One day in particular, in addition to this flow I felt exhausted but clear with the insight that my fatigue was related to the repression of various emotions that week. After I shared this with Dr. Chen, she helped me to understand that the two NSA entrainments that day allowed my sympathetic nervous system to finally take a break from supporting my mental judgment and resistance to my feeling full emotional expression. When my parasympathetic nervous system was finally able to kick in, it did so with so much force that I finally felt the exhaustion of ongoing emotional repression.

"You need to take care of yourself," Dr. Joyce reminded me. "Your soul is good. It's there! But you need to take care of yourself so that your soul can enter and share its message!"

Until that moment I was not aware of the direct relationship between a balanced nervous system and a safe and suitable home for my soul. Hearing about this relationship from a doctor I respected motivated me to take better care of myself for the sake of my true, authentic self—my soul.

In shedding masks layer by layer and reclaiming pieces of my soul, I am coming to learn that, like the evolving universe that I am a part of, my soul seeks to evolve its love and express its love. This to me is what spiritual transformation is.

It's interesting to note that the word "transformation" has the word "form" within it. Spirit requires the physical form of the human body so that it can transform. With no form, there is nothing to trans-form. Since healing requires feeling, with no physical form to feel, there is nothing to heal. From this spiritual perspective, I am able to perceive the human pains of life (or the first arrows, as the Buddha calls them) as opportunities to practise mindfulness and compassion. In doing so, I evolve my soul's love, transforming human pains into spiritual gains. The deeper into the darkness of my humanity I acknowledge, integrate, and heal, the more my love evolves and the brighter my soul's light shines outwards.

I find it beautiful that many cultures refer to the soul as being located in the centre of the chest, at the heart chakra. I've commonly heard the heart referred to as a burning fire, and this coincides with TCM knowledge that considers the heart to be of the element of fire. Fire is a powerful transformer, used to change matter into available energy, so it is an appropriate element to consider when transforming pain.

I actually have felt a real spark of fire in the centre of my chest only once in my life, but it was enough for me to believe that I do have an inner fire burning within me. This spark occurred in 2014 after I had visited my cousin and his wife in their new home. With the intention to help them with their new home, I hid money underneath one of their lamps. Knowing they had yet to furnish their place, I was confident they would find the money at some point in the near future. As I was walking down the stairs leaving their home, a vision came across my mind of the moment when they would find the money. Imagining the joy on their faces brought a joy to me, and with that feeling I felt and saw a spark inside my chest. Since this experience, I continue to fuel this inner fire with my breath. Sometimes when I am finding it very challenging to be with physical or emotional pain, I imagine myself holding the energies of the pains and then placing them in the transformative fire in my heart.

If Your Soul Wrote the Script to Your Life

While at the Omega Institute in New York, I was listening to Jon Kabat-Zinn provide a teaching around the mind-body connection, when one woman stood up and voiced a concern to the group. With tears in her eyes and a quiver in her voice, she shared her sense of confusion, anger, and guilt at the thought that she may have been the cause of her own cancer via her state of mind.

"Am I to blame for my own cancer?" she asked.

Jon Kabat-Zinn replied by saying that we should never let anyone allow us to feel like our conditions are our fault, for we are never wrong for having an illness or a pain condition. I did not fully comprehend what Jon was saying.

"With our minds affecting our bodies, are we not somehow contributing to our own illness with negative states of mind? Are we not fully responsible for how we allow our minds to affect our physical health?" I've asked myself in the past.

Since hearing that woman with cancer wonder about herself, I have been hesitant to answer this question with a yes, for it lays down the soil for self-blame and guilt to grow; and guilt is not something I want growing in the garden of my heart and mind.

One afternoon in the spring of 2017, when my medical qigong class had just completed its first clinical experience, I had the opportunity to explore this question again. I shared with my teacher and fellow classmates my concerns about the mind-body relationship and the potentially problematic perception that one is responsible for one's mind-body and thus possibly responsible for one's illnesses and pain. My teacher Wendy Lang gave an answer that broadened my perception of the mind-body connection to include that of the soul's purpose.

As with Jon's response, Wendy explained that we are never wrong or at fault for our illnesses and conditions. Instead of perceiving ourselves as victims and creators of our illnesses we can take an empowered view, acknowledging that the soul had a choice through which to experience this world. For instance, I'm coming to learn that my soul specifically chose me—the person called Jaisa Sulit—to experience this being human and evolve its love through specific lessons learned in this lifetime.

An interesting question Wendy posed to my classmates and me was "If life were a play, complete with its ups and downs, and a particular challenge such as cancer were a part of the story, what would the soul's purpose be for the cancer? How does cancer or another such challenge serve us? What would our soul want us to learn from the experience?"

I've gone on to share that question with others. One colleague who has fibromyalgia says that her fibromyalgia serves a purpose by reminding her to take care of herself better. Another colleague who has recovered from breast cancer says the cancer reminded her to love herself first. A close friend who had to go on bed rest for the last three months of her second pregnancy due to sacroiliac pain says the experience served as a reminder for her to ask others for help and to practise accepting things that she could not change. As for me, my accident and the pains that have unfolded since have served my healing and growth in so many ways that I too can't help but sometimes wonder, "Did my soul choose this accident so that I could evolve?"

With the spiritual world and its impacts on the physical body still being a mystery to many Western minds such as mine, I can only speculate on the causes and conditions for our accidents and illnesses. What I do know, though, is that the possibility that our souls may have chosen to experience specific challenges in order to serve our evolving love is a more empowering view than the belief that we are at fault and thus to blame for our illnesses.

No Longer Betraying My Own Soul

In her book *The Invitation*, Canadian storyteller and author Oriah "Mountain Dreamer" House says, "I want to know if you can disappoint another to be true to yourself. If you can bear the accusation of betrayal and not betray your own soul."[6]

For too long I've been on the cow path of wearing masks, silencing my inner voice, and sacrificing my soul's needs so as not to disappoint others. But when self-care is acknowledged as soul-care, then the betrayal of my personal needs becomes the betrayal of my soul's needs. This remembering that I have a role in helping my soul fulfill its purpose has made it easier for me to honour my needs, even at the risk of displeasing others. For instance, getting myself to finally express my soul's message through the publishing of this book required that I focus significantly more time on myself and less time on others. This meant that I finally had to learn to say no to family and close friends at the risk of the accusation of betrayal. Though it was initially scary for me, I've been learning to take those risks because I no longer want to betray my own soul.

I never used to believe in the concept of my soul reincarnating and thereby having multiple human lives. But with mindfulness, I am now conscious of the possibility that my soul has had previous lives. I can now acknowledge that this is my soul's first and only time to experience human living through this physical form of "Jaisa Sulit." This motivates me to take response-ability for my own soul-care by creating a safe space not only for my soul to reside but also for parts of my soul that have left to return, reinhabit, and remain. With a soul-care practice based on compassion and the attitudes of mindfulness such as non-judgment and beginner's mind, I am able to give my soul—my true, authentic self—the opportunity to fully experience the vividness that human living is meant to be. For when the time comes for my soul to move onward from this body, all it will take will be the moments met: the pleasant experiences, the unpleasant experiences, and everything in between. However the present moment is, experiencing it fully is what my soul needs.

Part IV

Experiencing the Mystery
of Spirit

12

Ghosts, Demons, and Past Lives, Oh My!

Facing Our Demons

"Welcome to Chinese Shamanic Medicine," were the words written on a flip chart at the front of the class.

"What the fuck? I didn't sign up for this," I thought to myself. It was the fall of 2016 and I was on the first day of my medical qigong course, or at least what I thought was medical qigong.

"I did not sign up for anything shamanic," I continued to think to myself. I did not know much about shamanism, nor was I interested in taking a course on it. Mysterious and unknown to me, shamanism frightened me. But I kept my judgments and fears to myself, until later that day when I had my first experience of witnessing an exorcism.

One of my classmates was experiencing menopause-like symptoms such as hot flashes and the feeling of something crawling on her skin. She was also in the middle of processing challenging emotions related to her relationship with her mother. Trusting and being open to healing, she courageously volunteered to have our teacher Wendy Lang work with her in front of the class for the sake of our collective learning. Wendy placed a chair in the centre of the room and had my classmate sit down.

"There are two demons here," Wendy said as she slowly walked around my classmate.

"What the fuck?" I thought to myself again. Until that point I never believed nor did I want to believe in the existence of demons. But I was intrigued and curious about what I was witnessing, so I continued to watch Wendy work.

Sharing with the class what her observations were, Wendy helped us to understand that two dark entities were feeding off my classmate's emotional energies. She went on to explain that everything, including humans, plants, animals, and even demons, has the thread of divine light within. But these demons (which is a common term many use to describe the dark, low-energy entities that exist in the spiritual realm) are so disconnected from the light within them that they need to feed off the divine light of other beings such as humans. When we get into moments when our emotions overwhelm and overcome us—such as my classmate was experiencing, being stuck in fear and worry—we end up giving these demons more energy to feed from. Interestingly for my classmate, one of the two demons actually belonged to her mother.

Now this exorcism was not the kind I have seen in movies; instead it looked more like what one would see in a psychotherapy room, where a therapist helps a client bring peace and understanding to an emotional dynamic with another person. In this case, however, the dynamic was with demons. Wendy facilitated a resolution between my classmate and the two demons, in which she was able to come to the understanding that the demons had a lesson for her to learn. By gaining insight into how she was unknowingly giving away her power, she was able to reclaim her power. Not only did my classmate end up thanking the demons for their role in her evolution, but with Wendy's help, she was also able to facilitate the demons' return to the divine light.

I wouldn't have believed what was happening in front of me if not for several of my classmates expressing how they sensed the lifting of a dark energy that turned into light. Also, after the demons had left, there was a consequent relaxation and calmness in my classmate's posture, with her face, neck, shoulders, and arms appearing to soften. When I asked her how she was doing, she expressed feeling lighter as if a weight had been lifted from her shoulders, the hot flashes had diminished, and the feeling of something crawling on her skin had disappeared.

Though a part of me was amazed at what I had seen, most of me was angry because I was confused and very uncomfortable. I raised my hand, and as soon as Wendy acknowledged me, I said, "What does all of this have to do with medical qigong? Why are we doing shamanic stuff? I don't even know if I want to believe in demons. I didn't sign up for this!"

Wendy responded by explaining that it was important everyone understood the history from which medical qigong has evolved. My classmates and I soon began to understand how all of the practices that have evolved from traditional Chinese medicine actually began with the practices developed by China's shamanic healers.

"Wow, I had no idea that traditional Chinese medicine had shamanic roots," I said to my classmate sitting beside me.

"Neither did I," she replied.

Honouring the shamanic context from which medical qigong has evolved, Wendy explained to my class that we had the option to complete additional training in channelling and mediumship, after which we would receive not only a practitioner certificate in medical qigong but also a practitioner certificate in Chinese shamanic medicine. When I heard that, I said to myself, "Hell, no. I am not going to get a shamanic certificate. My academic colleagues would think I'd gone nuts."

Our Ancestors Still Exist

Would you believe that within that same month I also witnessed numerous ancestral spirits enter the bodies of four of my colleagues? It was after this experience that I changed my mind and decided to take the channelling and mediumship courses and move forward with Chinese shamanic medicine.

I was at a Filipino-centred conference, where I was involved in gathering some items for an altar with the intention to honour our ancestors—both the ancestors of our Filipino lineage and the ancestors of the Squamish Nation, whose unceded lands we were holding the conference on. Growing up in a post-colonial culture, I had not inherited practices that acknowledged or reconnected me with my ancestors through my family's lineage. Consequently, I did not know what to expect at the conference. Nonetheless, I made sure I got the best of the local organic tobacco, rice, eggs, and salt, as these are apparently some of the ways to let the ancestors know we are honouring them with respect. Little did I know that our ancestors were actually going to come and visit us.

On the last day of this three-day conference, the majority of the conference attendees were gathered in one cabin, listening to a guest speaker from the United States. At the end of her talk she invited another guest speaker—Boi C—to approach the stage (*boi* means "female leader of a tribe," according to a particular indigenous group in the Philippines). When Boi C reached the front of the stage, the rest of the conference attendees were asked to direct their hands and attention toward her. After a few minutes of this directed attention toward Boi C, and with the guest speaker holding the space, Boi C dropped to the floor. When she stood up she started to speak with a different tone of voice.

"You are not listening," she said. I had spent some time speaking with Boi C throughout the three days at the conference, so I had a sense that it was not her but a spirit that was saying those words through her.

"You need to cleanse your hearts," the spirit said.

"Is this a possession?" I whispered to my friend Lea, who was standing next to me.

"I don't know!" she replied, with a look of fear in her eyes.

Boi C then fell to the floor again. Some of the conference leaders helped her up and brought her to lie beside the fireplace, where a fire had been burning 24-7 throughout the conference. Lea and I were called over to protect Boi C.

"I don't know what to do," Lea said to me with fear in her voice.

"I don't either," I replied.

We walked over to the fireplace, where Boi C was lying on a bench. Thankfully, there were several Filipino elders and healers and one Squamish healer present to guide us in how to protect ourselves. With Lea standing at Boi C's head and me at her feet, we held up a blanket to block spirits from returning to Boi C's body. But, as we stood there for the next hour, more spirits continued to arrive, and four other people in the cabin experienced having their bodies entered by ancestral spirits.

Continuing to guide us in self-protection, the elders and healers also engaged in communication with the arriving spirits. Apparently there were hundreds of them, all excited that people were now finally open to listening to what they've been wanting to tell us for so long. But the majority of us were not ready (myself included). We were not equipped with the knowledge systems and practices to connect safely with our ancestors. So with the help of the elders and healers in the room, we asked the spirits of our ancestors to be patient with us and leave us until we were ready to reconnect with them. The ancestors did listen and eventually left, and all those whose bodies were entered by spirit ended up recovering well.

I left the cabin that night with my beliefs blown apart.

"Wow. Our ancestors do still exist," I thought to myself as I walked back toward the sleeping lodge. Until that night I had been unaware of the possibility that I could access my ancestors. This insight into the continuity of my ancestral connections brought with it peace and gratitude in knowing that I now have another spiritual source to connect to in times of need. As I continue on my healing journey, I'm learning that not only are my ancestors still here for me but I can also now be here for them.

Carrying the Suffering of My Lineage

I've always heard of the notion that we carry our ancestors' suffering, through terms like "intergenerational trauma," but I didn't understand it on a personal level until I was at a Network Spinal Analysis (NSA) workshop called The Transformational Gate, developed and facilitated by chiropractor Donny Epstein, DC (also the creator of NSA). The workshop was held inside a large room with treatment tables formed in a circle; a dozen chiropractors provided NSA to approximately one hundred patients over the course of two days.

The energy of the large group was palpable, and I experienced a total of six powerful sessions at that workshop, each one leaving me with compounding improvements in posture and gait. But the most memorable session ended with me lying on the carpeted floor, overwhelmed with emotional pain. I was confused at the emotions I was feeling because they did not seem to be related to any particular situations in my life. The mix of anger, grief, and sadness was so overwhelming, I had to cry and wail very loudly just to release some of the energy. I was wailing so loudly that Dr. Epstein walked over to me from across the room. He knelt down, put one hand on my chest, paused for a few moments, and then said, "Honour the suffering of your lineage."

As soon as he acknowledged that the emotional pain I was experiencing was that of my ancestors, I felt a release within me. I felt a sense of peace in the understanding that the pain I was feeling was related to the suffering passed on through my bloodline. Epigenetics research describes how experiences are passed down through physical DNA in such a way that how my great-great-grandmother lived can affect my life now. But more meaningful than the passing on of painful experiences through our bloodline is the possibility that we can also pass on healing through the generations. My somato-experiencing practitioner Jane Courtney once shared with me the aboriginal wisdom that each decision we make affects the next seven generations, and the healing we do in this lifetime affects seven generations back and seven generations forward.

Now that I know my ancestors still exist and that I carry their suffering within my body, I am motivated more than ever to honour them by healing myself in this lifetime. I've been told that I can't heal my mother and my father, that I can only heal them by healing myself. How beautiful and hopeful is the possibility that in healing myself I heal the suffering of my predecessors, including my parents.

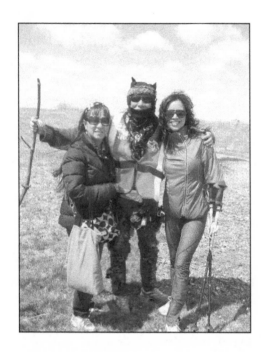

With my parents at the 2014 5k Walk for Multiple Sclerosis, which I was able to complete with the use of two hiking sticks, ankle foot orthoses, and orthotic arch supports.

Opening Up to the Unknown

I've always been afraid of the unseen. While I have a few friends who can connect with spiritual guides, angels, dead people, and even the spirits of plants and animals, I myself have always denied the reality of their existence. There was one instance in my childhood when a young girl saved me from drowning but, upon getting me to shore, she disappeared out of sight. Where did the girl go? Was she an angel? But I didn't believe in spiritual entities, let alone angels. Confused at what had happened, I didn't even bother to tell my parents that I had nearly drowned. From that day onward, I made myself believe that the girl who saved me was a fast runner who ran away soon as she'd brought me to shore.

But after witnessing the existence of ancestral spirits at the Filipino-centred conference, I became motivated to take the channelling and mediumship courses that Wendy Lang spoke of at our first day of class. I felt I would be powerless in my ability to help those whose bodies were entered by spirits and used as channels without that training. I also felt incapable of connecting with the ancestral spirits who clearly wanted to communicate with us. With a desire to be of better service the next time a situation like that were to happen, I got over my judgments and fears of the unseen and completed one course in mediumship and two courses in channelling.

Channelling: Connecting with My Guides

I was initially scared to practise channelling because I grew up believing that any spiritual practice not involving Jesus Christ specifically is of the devil. For instance, I've been judged by some for partaking in yoga and meditation, with statements such as "Jesus did not teach yoga or meditation."

So when the time came for me to attempt my first channelling experience, I was filled with fear. "What if I channel something evil?" I thought to myself.

Fortunately, I trusted Wendy Lang and her ability to create and hold safe and sacred spaces. I also found comfort in the channelling and mediumship processes that Wendy teaches, because they are always grounded in the will of the divine and the highest good of all; to my Catholic-conditioned mindset, that sounds the same as God's will, so I felt safe to move forward with the learning experience.

The required reading for the channelling course was the book *Opening to Channel: How to Connect with Your Guide* by Sanaya Roman and Duane Packer.[7] I was very surprised at how simple the channelling process seemed to be. The channelling class had about twenty-five people, many of whom were healthcare professionals. The Newtonian-thinking part of me found validation that I was not in a group with "weird" people. But before we moved on to connecting with our guides, we first practised connecting with rocks and plants.

"Oh my gosh. Listening to a rock?" I thought. I was officially becoming one of the "weird" people I was afraid I would be among that day. I could not believe we were going to attempt listening to a plant, let alone a rock.

Everyone was given a different type of rock and, surprisingly, everyone—including me—was able to connect with the spirit of their rock and receive its message. The rock I was holding gave me the message that it was sad it had been taken away from its ecosystem but was happy to be of service in a different way through its contribution to the channelling course.

Similarly for the next exercise, each person was given a leaf or a branch that they were to connect to. To my surprise, again everyone was able to connect and receive the message of what they were holding. I couldn't believe it, and I found validation from others around me who also couldn't believe it. But collectively, we could not deny our inner sense of knowing that we each felt connected to the spirits of the rocks and the plants. It was a great practice in connecting to our own sense of intuition, a skill needed to connect with one's guides.

Having first cultivated a greater sense of trust in our intuition, we moved forward, working in pairs, and attempted to connect with our spiritual guides. I was amazed, because everyone in the class—including myself, again—was able to connect with at least one guide.

Since that course I have continued to develop my own practice of channelling my highest spiritual guides whenever I need wise counsel. Though there was much doubt in the beginning as to whether I really was connecting with my guides or whether it was all in my imagination, with ongoing practice and the sharing of my practice with friends who also practise channelling, I have been gaining more confidence in my ability to connect with the highest guides, who help me to live in alignment with my soul's purpose and the highest good of all.

Mediumship: Connecting with Dead People

Although I easily overcame my fear of connecting with my guides, I was more afraid of connecting with dead people. High guides are always loving and compassionate, whereas dead people are not always so. But as she does with all her courses, Wendy Lang created a space that made everyone feel safe to explore the experience of being a medium. During her two-day mediumship course, eight other people and I learned how to connect with people who have passed. As with the channelling course, initially we practised just learning how to trust our intuition and inner knowing. Unlike in the channelling course, where we connected with guides in pairs, in the mediumship course we always worked in groups of three or more. I liked that because it made me feel comfortable to have more people connecting with the same dead person I was attempting to connect with. Some people were much better at mediumship than others; I was definitely not one of the better ones.

While I enjoyed channelling guides more than I did trying

to be a medium for dead people, I came out of that course with an appreciation for the role of mediumship in our health and wellness. For instance, with the help of three other people in that class, we were able to connect with my grandmother, who had passed away in 1998. My grandmother had spent her last few years living in a nursing home. My mother and I have always carried guilt for placing her in a nursing home, because she did not want to be there. However, due to her dementia and her need for twenty-four-hour supervision, which my family was unable to provide, we felt we had no choice. Despite forgiving ourselves, my mom and I have never really been at peace with my grandmother's passing away alone in a nursing home. However, with the opportunity to finally connect with her in the mediumship class, I apologized to my grandmother. I myself did not have any sense of her in the room, but the other three people in my group were able to sense her and relayed her messages to me. With their help I was able to get answers to questions such as how she was not mad at all for being placed in the nursing home and was apparently very ready to go when she did. It brought me peace to know that, unlike some others who have passed, my grandmother was resting in peace.

Apparently she continues to watch over me, providing me with guidance when I need it. Furthermore, all three people in my group were able to sense a young male presence beside her. Upon speaking to my mom and uncle about this, I learned for the first time that my grandmother actually had another son, who had died in his youth. Most likely this male presence standing beside my grandmother was my mom and uncle's brother. It makes me happy to think that not only is my grandmother not upset with my mom and me but she is resting in peace in the company of one of her children.

Connecting with Past Lives

Growing up Catholic, I didn't acknowledge the existence of my past lives and how they can affect my health and wellness in this current life—until I took the medical qigong practitioner program. At the end of the program, my classmates and I had to complete a two-day clinic where volunteer patients would be able to receive our medical qigong healing sessions. During these two days, my classmates and I were paired up with qigong masters who, with their many more years of experience, could provide us practitioners with mentorship.

I still clearly remember the first patient my partner and I worked with. Let's call the patient Jen. Jen came in with complaints of shoulder pain and fatigue. After my partner and I spent some time interviewing her and explaining what we would be doing, we asked Jen to get on the table and we began to work. During that session, we discovered that not only was Jen's grandmother raped and the trauma passed on to Jen, but Jen herself had been a Japanese warrior who killed and raped others in a previous lifetime. Jen was able to see the karmic balance in being both the one who raped others in a past life and the one who had been raped, via her lineage through her grandmother.

This warrior had a powerful ability to use the element of fire and used it to cause harm. Though the physical body of the warrior was gone, its spirit still carried with it much guilt, a guilt that had continued to be carried within Jen in this lifetime. Jen said that up until this session for many years she had felt unable to breathe into her belly, as if she were not allowed to breathe deeply. My partner then guided a dialogue between Jen and this warrior spirit until Jen realized that this warrior's guilt was the reason she had been unknowingly disallowing herself to breathe fully, so as to suppress the fire inside her. With my partner's continued compassionate guidance Jen was able to thank the warrior for giving her the power of fire and facilitate the warrior spirit's return to divine light.

When Jen sat up from the table, she began to cry. Not only had the shoulder pain disappeared, she felt full of energy. "I'm reclaiming the power of my inner fire and am excited to use it to serve others," she said.

What unfolded on the table with Jen that day has not only taught me to be open to the possibility that past lives can affect how I feel in this current life, but that in the grand scheme of all my lives, I may have been both the good and the bad, both the victim and the villain, both the marginalized and the oppressor, and both the healer and the harmer. Wendy Lang said once in class, "True compassion has to come out of humility," because all of our souls have been to "dark and dirty places."

Allowing this possibility to exist within my awareness helps me come to a sense of balance, harmony, and peace in the midst of the pain and suffering that has always existed in this world.

13

Connecting with Her Spirit

No Earth—No Qigong

Medical qigong has rebirthed my connection to Mother Earth, because it is a practice that requires working with and balancing the energies of both yang and yin. For instance, medical qigong has me connecting regularly with the masculine yang energies of the sun and the stars, which many of our indigenous communities refer to as Father Sky. I also connect daily with the feminine yin energies of the earth, accordingly referred to as Mother Earth.

This being said, with no earth there is no yin to balance the yang. No earth—no qigong.

Now, connecting with the existence of qi and my soul within me has been one thing, but the discovery of qi and spirit within rocks, plants, and animals has been another. Many indigenous communities believe that all things, including plants and animals, are animated by a life force or spirit, and "animism" is the anthropological construct used to describe these beliefs. For most of my life, I've judged these animistic beliefs negatively, terming them "pagan," so it was not until I was almost at the end of my medical qigong practitioner training that I really shed my colonial-conditioned judgments and began to reclaim my innate connection to Mother Earth and her guiding spirit.

Guidance from Plants and Trees

During one of my medical qigong practitioner classes in the spring of 2017, my classmates and I were each to bring in two glass dropper bottles so that we could learn how to make plant essences. Never having made plant essences before, I asked one of the teaching assistants, "When are we going to be picking flowers?"

"We are not going to be picking anything," she replied, to my surprise.

I was so confused. How in the world were we going to make plant essences without plucking anything out from the ground? Later that afternoon, we each filled our glass dropper bottles with the same ratio of water and alcohol. We were then to go outside and, with our developing intuition, we were to discern which plants were calling out to us.

I could not believe what I was going to attempt to do, but with curiosity leading the way, I went on with the activity despite the fear of judgment should anyone see me communicating with plants. Note: our classes were held inside Vancouver's Stanley Park, so there were always people around; I anticipated having strangers staring at me, thinking I was cuckoo.

I was to make one bottle of a plant essence for myself and the other bottle for a classmate, who was represented by a number that I had pulled out of a hat. Since I did not know who I was making the second plant essence for, I could only guess who the bottle was for based on the messages I received from the plants that called to me.

For the first bottle, which was for me, I walked around the park trying to listen and feel out any sense of pull to a particular plant or tree. After walking around for five minutes, I ended up under a large conifer tree. Standing beneath the tree I felt a sense of being very grounded, centred, and strong, and standing very tall with confidence and wisdom. As instructed by my teacher, I asked the tree if it would allow me to work with it. Surprisingly, I got a sense of it saying yes, through a feeling in my body that felt safe and held with love. I then began to pull its energy in through my left hand and direct its flow up my left arm, across my upper torso, down my right arm, and into the bottle that I was holding in my right hand. I continued to fill the water-alcohol solution with the tree's energy until the tree gave me a sign to stop. The tree's message to stop came to me as a sense of inner knowing. I then asked the tree to tell me the recommended dosage of the plant essence. Again, through the sense of inner knowing, I received the message to intake only one drop of the solution as needed.

Once I was done with my personal bottle, I moved on to work with other plants and trees to make a plant essence for my mystery classmate. I approached more trees, various flowers, and bushes, until ten minutes later I felt a pull toward one tall flower and one particular deciduous tree. The flower gave me the message to be strong and courageous in leadership, to have a beautiful mind, and to use intuition. The deciduous tree gave me the message to be grounded in divine connection and made me feel safe and protected. I worked with the flower and the deciduous tree as I had with the conifer tree, pulling its energy in through my left hand, directing its flow up my left arm, across my upper torso, down my right arm, and into the bottle in my right hand. I filled the solution with energy until I sensed the message to stop. After working with both the flower and the deciduous tree, I asked for the recommended dosages.

"Take one drop as needed until the bottle is empty," was

the message I received, though I still had some doubt that I might be making things up.

"Am I really communicating with trees now?" I thought to myself with a growing sense of excitement.

As I walked back to class with my two bottles of plant essences, I tried to think which mystery classmate my second bottle was for. Based on the messages and the feelings of the essences in the bottle, I had a gut instinct as to who in the class would benefit from this. Lo and behold, once the mystery names were revealed to us, it was amazing how not only was my own guess correct, but so were the guesses of all my classmates.

The really surprising part for me occurred when I tasted the solution in the bottle that I made for myself and compared it with the taste of the essences that one of my classmates made for me. The taste was significantly different, with one tasting as though it had double the amount of vodka. How could that be, when everyone received the same solution mixture of water and alcohol from the same bottle? I could only attribute it to the different plant essences that were put into the bottle by each practitioner.

Guidance from Animals

It was not until my experience with the shaman at the Omega Institute that I was introduced to the concept of acknowledging the spirits of animals as a form of medicine. Displayed on the walls of the shaman's healing space were images of various types of animals, but it was the deer that I was immediately drawn to. The shaman told me that *deer* must be my spirit animal. I was quite happy with that, because with thousands of deer living in Ontario, it is not uncommon for me to see deer when I spend time outside Toronto. However, every now and then the image of a deer will appear in my mind, in my dreams, or in a magazine. Whether a deer appears to me in physical form or in a mental-spiritual form, it always comes at a perfect time, when I need to be reminded by its message to pause, bring awareness to the moment, connect with my innate dignity, and hold my head up with grace.

A few years after being introduced to the guidance of deer, a friend gifted me with a set of cards called *Medicine Cards: The Discovery of Power through the Ways of Animals* by Jamie Sams, David Carson, and Angela C. Werneke. It is a method of divination that helps each soul find its path via the ancient medicine of animals.

"Are these like tarot cards?" I thought to myself with feelings of fear; I grew up considering tarot cards to be evil. Consequently, I was initially hesitant to use the Medicine Cards. However, within the same year of receiving the cards I was gifted with a second set of the same cards from a different friend. I took it as a sign to be curious and to open up to exploring the cards in my life.

The first Medicine Card spread that I completed was that of the nine totem animals, where a different totem animal provides me with guidance for each direction, including east, south, west, north, above, below, and within, as well as my left side and my right side (each direction corresponding to a different aspect of my life). To demonstrate the benefit of animal medicine, let's take for example the direction within. The animal guiding the direction within is said to teach us how to protect our sacred space and how to be faithful to our personal truths. The totem animal guiding my direction within is the prairie dog, whose medicine teaches me to retreat into stillness in order to replenish my life force and find strength and inspiration. To this day, whenever I pull the prairie dog card or see a prairie dog in my dreams, it is always during a time when I need a reminder to rest and retreat.

Since completing the nine-totem-animal spread, I've continued to use the Medicine Cards, whether it be via a multi-card spread, the pulling of one card, or returning to my nine totem animals. Over time, my sense of connection to and trust in the guidance of animals and their spirits has deepened. I've also gone on to use other divination cards to connect with the guiding spirit of Mother Earth, such as *Gaia Oracle: Guidance, Affirmations, Transformation* by Toni Carmine Salerno. Whether I use the animal medicine cards or the *Gaia Oracle* cards, the wisdom of Mother Earth, her plants, trees, and animals, continues to be another resource that I can now trust and rely on as a resource for strength, wisdom, and love.

Even in the City

I am very fortunate to have had the opportunity to befriend Boi C, who is not only a tribal leader but a shamanic healer as well. Her tribe lives on the foot of Mount Apo, a stratovolcano that is the tallest mountain in the Philippines. There, where she lives on the lands of her ancestors in the midst of Mother Nature, she is able to connect easily with the guidance of spirit. But whenever she is in a metropolitan city, she needs to use playing cards to interpret messages from spirit. By establishing a code where each playing card has a different meaning, she has created her own divination process.

While the use of divination cards can help us to interpret more precisely the guidance of divine spirit, living back in a metropolis such as Toronto is teaching me that spirit is creative and has infinite ways to guide me, with or without the use of cards.

Since opening up to the guiding spirit of Mother Earth, I have been visited more often by animals in my dreams and meditations. When I left Vancouver for Toronto, I was initially scared that I would lose my connection to Mother Earth. But since my return, I've learned that no matter where I live, Mother Earth is always beneath my feet. Though it is more challenging to connect with her spirit in the city, it has not been impossible, but it does require that I listen and pay attention more deeply.

Deepening Relations with Her

As my relationship with Mother Earth becomes more intimate, I find myself connecting more with other women who are in conscious relationship with Mother Earth and her spirit. One of these women is Corrine Enojo, who has allowed me to share one of her dreams in this book. In the dream I'm about to share with you, Corrine is given a message of how one is to greet the land upon which one arrives.

During the first three steps, one is to greet the land and introduce one's self. During the next three steps, one is to think about what one knows about the land, and during the final three steps, one is to think about and share the type of relationship one wants to build with the land from this time forward.

I explored this way of greeting the land upon my return to Toronto. When I got off the plane, I greeted the land as guided by Corrine's dream. I introduced myself and greeted the land, reminding myself that "Toronto" is a name derived from the Mohawk word *tkaronto*, meaning "trees standing in the water" or "trees by the water." Before learning of Tkaronto's traditional name, I had no idea that Toronto was an area where trees grew in shallow water. I then took some moments to acknowledge the indigenous communities that lived and continue to live here and how little I actually knew of the history of Tkaronto pre-colonization. I then went on to share with the land my intentions to deepen my relationship with her through the practice of daily connection and listening, to explore the practice of reconciliation, and finally, to educate others on her direct role in our health and healing.

While it took more than nine steps for me to complete this way of greeting the land, it took me less than five minutes to do so (and I was still far from reaching baggage claim). Though brief, I found this a meaningful practice that grounded me and forced me to reflect, expand my awareness, and cultivate intentionality. Since that day I have felt a deeper connection to the land, waters, and animals of Tkaronto, which brings with it a sense of being listened to and supported, as well as a sense of responsibility to her.

Supported by the Spirit of Stawamus Chief Mountain

In the spring of 2017, I achieved my greatest physical and mental feat yet, and it was not without the help of spiritual connection. With assistance from the Canadian Adaptive Climbing Society, a project founded by Brent Goodman, I climbed to the top of the Apron, which is approximately 350 feet high and is considered one of the classic routes on the famous Stawamus Chief Mountain. Located in Squamish, British Columbia, Stawamus Chief Mountain is one of the largest granite monoliths in the world, and is referred to by some as The Chief.

Considering I have such limited tolerance for standing and walking, it still boggles my mind as to how I was able to scale the granite face of The Chief. Throughout the climb there were many moments when it appeared as though my body was giving out and I couldn't even stand on my feet anymore. During those moments, I would apply what I learned in medical qigong class and expand my awareness to include my physical, energetic, and spiritual bodies. Every time I connected with all three bodies I felt a second wind. However, there was one moment in particular when I was feeling tired and full of doubt. I was halfway up to the top of the Apron, when I thought about giving up and just being satisfied with how far I had gotten. But then I remembered that the climb was not just for me—it was for the Canadian Adaptive Climbing Society and the people whom that group serves. Getting to the top would have meaning not just for me but possibly for others who might find inspiration in my getting to the top. So in those moments of desperation, I dug deeper than I ever had in my life. I connected deep within my core and deep into the core of Stawamus Chief Mountain. I expanded my awareness of my spiritual body until I felt one with her spirit, and I asked her to help me.

What I'm about to say is so unbelievable that I have some doubt about it myself. After I connected with the spirit of Stawamus, not only did I get a rush of energy to continue climbing, but it was as if Stawamus was helping me up her granite face herself. There were so many times when I felt like my foot was going to slip, and a crack, bump, or ledge seemed to protrude from the rock face, giving me solid footing.

"Is this really happening?" I thought to myself each time my foot found solid purchase despite it seeming as though there would be nothing to step up from.

As if one were to walk on water and trust that a rock was underneath the water's surface with every step, I kept moving upward, finding places for my feet to step on. After eleven pitches, six hours of climbing, and a lot of encouragement from Brent and mountain guide Ian Middleton, I was able to get my body to the top of the Apron.

Before rappelling down the side of the mountain, I took some time to enjoy the view, celebrate, and reflect. I felt at peace. There was a new sense of awe and respect for Stawamus Chief Mountain. Also, I had a deeper sense of trust in the love and support of her spirit.

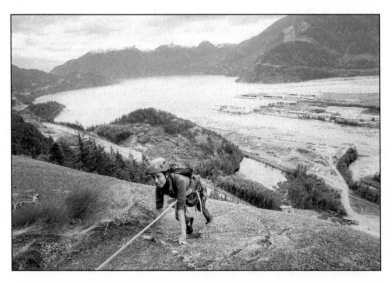

Climbing Stawamus Chief Mountain on June 7, 2017 with the help of the Canadian Adaptive Climbing Society, almost seven years after the accident.

14

Returning to Wholeness

I Became Everything

When perceiving reality through a set of lenses that acknowledges only the physical world, it appears we are separate from each other. But from the perspective of a broader set of lenses that includes energetic and spiritual realities, it becomes easier to conceive our interconnectedness in oneness, or in other words, how we are all part of one whole.

I have had varying experiences of this mysterious yet undeniable sense of our unity—all of them always when I am in solitude and in silence, meditating with compassion. For instance, in the summer of 2013 I joined Satipanna Insight Meditation Toronto in their seven-day Vipassana and Metta Meditation Retreat at Chapin Mill Retreat Center in Batavia, New York. Unlike the S. N. Goenka retreat, where the majority of one's meditation practice is done inside a meditation hall, Satipanna Insight teachers Jim Bedard and Randy Baker offered a schedule that allowed some time each day for meditators to practise anywhere, including outside in nature. Located on a 135-acre property in the countryside, Chapin Mill offered me the opportunity to extend my awareness to the skies above me, the earth beneath me, the waters before me, and a diversity of plants, trees, birds, and insects around me. Each day I would find a new place outside in nature to meditate on *metta*, which means "loving kindness" in Pali (the ancient language used widely in Buddhist literature).

On the sixth day of practice, while meditating on the feeling of my breathing body and extending *metta* outwards, something bizarre happened. All of a sudden, I felt as though I was an expanding cloud of light that grew to encompass the air around my body, the trees, the earth beneath me, the pond in front of me, and even the sky above me, including the birds flying by.

I was becoming everything.

Confused at what was occurring to me, I opened my eyes and looked around me. I was still in my body. I was still sitting on my cushion.

"What just happened?" I thought to myself. "And why does this feel familiar?"

It then dawned on me that I had experienced something similar the year before, while I was at the Scandinave Spa in Vieux-Montréal. I had spent a whole day at that spa, treating myself to a full body massage and multiple cycles through the sauna, the hot tub, the cold-water plunge, and the relaxation beds. Throughout my time at the spa, whether I was in the water, on the massage table, or resting on a relaxation bed, I committed to doing a body scan. At the end of that day, after my last water-therapy cycle, I lay down on a bench and continued with a body scan. My body felt very relaxed and my mind was calm and fully focused on my body. All of a sudden, I started to experience everything going bright, and I no longer felt my physical body lying on the bench. I felt as though I was an expanding warm light that was encompassing the entire space within the room, all the way up to the ceiling.

Scared, I immediately opened my eyes and sat up.

"Did I just faint?" I thought to myself.

But I had fainted before and it was a very different experience, where everything goes black, not bright. Furthermore, with fainting I experience losing my sense of awareness, but with this expansive experience my sense of awareness was growing.

I didn't tell anyone of this experience at the Scandinave Spa because I didn't think anyone would be able to relate or validate what had happened. I almost forgot about it until the similar experience happened at Chapin Mill.

My most recent experience of becoming one with everything happened in the summer of 2017, during a meditation on the beach after doing medical qigong. I was sitting barefoot on a log, feet connected to the earth beneath me and my compassionate awareness reaching out deep into the core of the earth and up above to the sun, moon, stars, and planets. All of a sudden, for a brief moment, I felt as if my body had become a part of the universe. My experience of the physical body disappeared and instead I saw a bright sun in the centre of my being, and all around it was a vast darkness with an infinite number of stars.

"Wow. As above so below," I thought to myself upon opening my eyes. "I am in the universe yet the universe is within me!"

While these experiences of feeling connected to the vastness of everything have always been brief, they have been enough for me to remember who I really am and what I am not. I am love, and everything else is an opportunity for me to express that which I am.

It's All Love

Growing up, I learned to put God in a box, with the belief that I completely understood this mysterious divine. I even assigned

"Him" a gender, dismissing the feminine aspect of divinity altogether. After years of trying to intellectualize the divine, I've come to accept that I can't logically understand the ways of the mysterious spiritual world. I love the God I was raised to connect with, but I also love learning about the Dharma and the Dao; several of my teachers have told me "It's all the same." Whether this greatest spiritual mystery is referred to as the Universe, our Collective Consciousness, the Absolute, the Great Spirit, the Source, or the Creator of all things, one thing that I know for sure is that it's all love.

During that seven-day Vipassana and Metta Retreat at Chapin Mill in 2013 (where I experienced becoming everything), I was outdoors doing a walking meditation when I started to feel pain in my feet and back. I sat down on a bench to rest, and because I had been cultivating curious accepting awareness all week, I welcomed an emerging wave of energy that was starting to well up from my chest into my throat. Next thing I knew, I began to bawl and wail out loud. As the tears flowed, all I felt was grief and sorrow for the physical and functional abilities I had lost and the physical and emotional pains I had gained in return. I wasn't feeling pity or sorrow for myself, but instead I felt a raw sadness for all the hardship and struggle I had gone through up until that point yet had never acknowledged or honoured.

A few minutes later, I became overwhelmed with a feeling of being heard and held with love. I looked up and around me, and I experienced a surreal sense of the trees listening to me, the birds listening to me, the grass, the pond, the flowers, and the sky—all were listening to me. I experienced a sense of comfort in my pains being acknowledged and held with compassion.

I felt intimately seen, heard, and loved.

A similar experience happened to me while on a silent retreat at the Manresa Jesuit Spiritual Renewal Centre in Pickering, Ontario, that same year. I was doing a mindful walking meditation within an outdoor labyrinth. When I got to the centre, I paused to do a standing meditation. While standing there breathing, all of a sudden I became filled with an energy that was comforting and compassionate. This oncoming energy guided my arms and hands upward to a position of hugging myself.

"Am I doing this?" I thought to myself with bewilderment as I observed my arms moving not of my own volition but because of a force that felt much greater than me. It was a force that made me feel connected, safe, loved, and held with compassion.

I stood there in the centre of the labyrinth with my arms wrapped around myself for a minute or so. It was a magical moment because it did not feel like I was the one hugging myself—I felt like I was being hugged by God.

I Am Never Alone

Perhaps the most dramatic experience I've had of being loved by a mysterious force was in 2012, two years after my accident. I was in my bedroom sitting cross-legged on my bed in the dark, caught in a mental tornado of fear. At that point I had been single for one year. From 1998 until 2011, I went from one boyfriend to the next so I had never been single even for one day.

I was afraid to be alone.

Since the accident I also had more anxiety about my parents unexpectedly dying.

"When they die, I'll have no one!" I was thinking to myself

that night. I even called my friend Mayleen to let her know that when my parents were both gone I would move near her so that I wouldn't be alone.

After I got off the phone with Mayleen I continued to sit on my bed in the dark by myself. At some point, I somehow got the courage to face my fear of being alone and opened my mind and heart to fully feel the fear. Suddenly I sensed a dark cloudlike presence appear in the room. The more I cried in fear of facing a potential future of being alone, the bigger the cloud grew and the darker it became. As I moved deeper into the darkness of my fears, I eventually approached what has felt like the darkest and lowest moment in my life, when all of a sudden I met God.

I felt loved.

It was love.

I was part of it and it was a part of me.

In those moments of connection, I finally understood that I am never alone.

It's That Thing

To express my experiences of connection to the mystery of the divine, I wrote "That Thing," the spoken word piece that I shared at the Roots Lounge Open Mic and Poetry Slam in Toronto. It continues to be my favourite poem that I've written yet.

That Thing
Ahh, the journey within.
Of all paths taken
Nothing has been more painful
Yet beautiful and worthwhile
Than the path to self-love

Why, oh why
Has it been easier for me to show more love to others than to
myself?
But that thing
As I venture closer
Closer to the space within
I feel that thing

Call it God
Call it Light
Call it Love
Call it Life
It's the Force
It's the Universe
It's that thing

It's that thing that makes me feel that I am one
One with him
One with her
One with you
One with life

It's connecting to that thing
That makes loving myself come so naturally.
It's connecting to that thing
That makes accepting myself unconditionally just the thing to
do.

How good it feels to finally BE REAL

REAL!

Two sides to the coin
This journey
This journey that has brought me to the depths of darkness

Pain
Reality
Bringing me closer
Closer to that thing
Where when the seasons change and the tides seem too
strong
It's that thing inside me deep within
That is like a stable rock

It's where I find peace
It's where I find love

It's when I connect to that thing
That instead of falling apart
Life falls into place

Instead of closing in
Life is unfolding
And instead of resisting
Life is just flowing

How complex this journey is
And yet
So simple
It's as simple as breathing.

It's with every breath
Every inhale
And every exhale
In
Out
I connect
I connect to that thing

I connect to that thing within me and within you
In
Out
We connect

We connect to that thing

That thing

Remembering that I am part of "that thing" has helped me bring perspective to challenging times. For instance, when I observe myself back on a cow path, engaging in a judgmental pattern, I find comfort in remembering that I am more than these habitual patterns. I am more than this physical body and the sensations of pain, and I am more than these fleeting thoughts and emotions. I am part of a loving force that is greater than any form of pain. So, more than anything, I am the loving awareness of these human experiences.

Discovering Our Interconnectedness through Distance Healing

The concept of wholeness and oneness was easier for me to

conceive after I opened up to experiencing distance healing. For it was in the receiving and giving of energy healing from a distance that I realized the truth of our interconnectedness. While living in Vancouver with all of my family still in Toronto, I began to explore providing reiki and medical qigong healing sessions from a distance. Though I had initial doubts about the effectiveness of my distance sessions, the feedback I would receive from the person receiving my sessions only validated that what I was doing was really causing a palpable and beneficial effect.

"How is it possible that the mental intentions and physical actions that I am engaging in in one area of the country can result in palpable changes in sensation and emotion in the person I am working on, who is on the other side of the country?" I would ask myself.

"How is it possible that I am actually able to sense into how someone far away is feeling, physically and emotionally?" I'd wonder.

Several of my therapists in Toronto also made it known to me that we would be able to continue our work together from a distance while I lived in Vancouver. I was initially doubtful. How can somebody who is three time zones, four provinces, and a five-hour flight away from me affect my body and mind? But whether the distance session was in the form of reiki, BodyTalk, or Reconnective Healing, I always experienced more relaxation, less pain, improved body awareness, improved mood, and greater insight after each session. I was surprised to discover that distance sessions were no less beneficial than in-person sessions.

It turns out distance healing is possible because of our interconnectedness as one whole.

Science Supports Our Wholeness

Quantum physicists state quantum entanglement is the mechanism for our interconnectedness and ability to provide energy healing from a distance. "Quantum entanglement" is a term used to describe the physical phenomenon in which the activities of entangled particles correlate with each other even when large distances separate the particles from each other. Quantum entanglement points to the notion that instead of individual particles being independent of each other, they are actually part of a whole system in which each individual particle is interconnected. While the science supporting our interconnectedness is recent, the notion of it is ancient, through spiritual teachers such as Jesus and the Buddha, who referred to our oneness in their teachings.

Considering we are interconnected as one whole, it makes sense that what I do unto others I do unto myself and vice versa. When I judge and harm myself, I inadvertently cause harm to everyone else that I am interconnected with. But when I heal myself, I also bring healing to the wholeness that I am part of. This truth of our interconnectedness is what inspires me to embrace physical and emotional pain as opportunities for learning and growth, for when I gain, the whole gains.

It's Not About Me

There is a reason why there is the word "we" in wellness and the word "I" in illness. I discovered that during my first Vipassana meditation retreat in 2012. On the last day of the ten-day retreat, while watching a video recording of S. N. Goenka, a truth hit me like a truck. An insight arose within me, a sense of knowing that was so clear that my body instantly felt lighter.

"Compassion! 'Com-passion' is community passion," I thought to myself with joy.

During the retreat I observed how so much of my mind's attention was focused on my book, my story, my journey, and what other people thought about me. Seeing my mind from an observer's point of view made it apparent to me that I was causing my own misery by worrying about myself all the time.

"It's not about me!" I discovered.

"It's about compassion for community!"

The enlightenment of that truth was physically palpable as I walked out of the meditation hall, feeling lighter; everything around me seemed more vibrant and clear. The sky was more blue, the trees were more green, and the sun appeared to be shining more brightly. I felt a sense of peace and trust in the truth I had just embodied.

We Are Each Other's Medicine

In contemplating our interconnectedness as one spiritual community, it becomes apparent that healing unfolds when we gather together as a community in safe spaces, spaces that are judgment-free and compassionate. For centuries, our ancestors lived in villages where friends and families could easily gather together to eat, tell stories, make music, and dance, and this provided a regularly needed space for connection and healing. Though I do not live in one physical village with all my friends and family, I have been able to experience the medicine of a compassionate community through the opportunity to take part in different kinds of healing circles.

Seeing Self in Other

One such circle is a three-month therapeutic writing group facilitated by Melissa Melnitzer, MD, which I enjoyed so much I completed it twice. Dr. Melnitzer is a family physician in Toronto who facilitates weekly sessions that are two hours and fifteen minutes in length. Every session begins with approximately forty-five minutes of journaling on the topic of that week. Examples of topics include "If I loved myself enough. Write about how well you can take it. Write about a relationship," and "Write about a time you felt beautiful." After this journaling period, Dr. Melnitzer then guides the group in a meditation. The rest of the session is a facilitated discussion, when participants have the opportunity to read aloud what they wrote in their journal.

While I found healing in the process of writing, I was surprised to experience even more healing in the reading of my writing to my fellow group participants. There were a good handful of times when, as I was reading, all of a sudden I broke out in tears. There was a significant difference between expressing myself silently to a journal and expressing myself aloud to a group. Though I felt more vulnerable, the witnessing of my expressions with non-judgment and compassion made me feel acknowledged in a way that journaling cannot.

The other circle that I was part of was a mindfulness-for-chronic-pain group that meets once a month at Bridgepoint Active Healthcare. Many people with chronic pain often feel alone, isolated, and misunderstood, because chronic pain is one of those invisible disabilities where those who don't experience it can't really understand the daily struggle. So whenever this group gets together each month to sit in a circle of mindfulness and compassion, there is always the same sigh of relief in the validation of our emotions and the remembering that we are not alone in our suffering. Furthermore, because this was not just a chronic-pain group but a mindfulness chronic-pain group, it was such a gift to meet each month and see how mindfulness was continuing to be beneficial. But what was even more helpful was seeing how common it was for people to fall off the wagon. To know we were not alone in our struggle to maintain a daily mindfulness practice when "life got busy" made it easier for each of us to accept our humanity. We each understood that struggling with our daily practice is both normal and okay.

My experiences in both the therapeutic writing group and the monthly mindfulness-for-chronic-pain group have taught me that healing arises when we allow our human emotions to be witnessed by others. Because we are all part of the same whole, when we witness another person's emotional expressions, we are also witnessing a part of ourselves in them. Just as you may see a part of yourself in my story, I may see a part of myself in your story too, no matter how different we may be.

In each other, we see ourselves.

In the Philippines we actually have a word to describe this concept. The word *kapwa* is used to refer to "our shared identity, our shared inner self" or our sense of "self in other." So when we gather in compassionate community to honestly share our experiences of joy, pain, and suffering, we experience *kapwa*. Just as we see that part of ourselves that suffers when we witness another person's suffering, the beauty of *kapwa* is that we can also experience a part of ourselves healing when we witness each other's healing. For instance, after reading my journal entry during one of the therapeutic writing sessions, I was approached by one group participant who shared how a part of her was able to heal in witnessing me. She said that she no longer knew how to cry, but in seeing me cry, she was able to experience a catharsis for her repressed emotions.

I'm Not That Unique!

Mindfulness has helped me to discover that a lot of my stress, anxiety, and depression have arisen from the need to be unique and different from everyone else. I especially started to feel this stress when I became self-employed and had to start defining my brand. One problem with branding is there's this need to set oneself apart, to be special, different, and unique. Paradoxically, that's the opposite of what I have really needed. With a judgmental mind that defines my being based on being different from others, I am also sending myself the message that my problems, my pain, and my suffering are also different from others'. The belief that my habits of self-loathing and self-doubt, my fears and my worries, are unique to me makes me feel depressed and alone in my misery, but the gift of being able to witness the sufferings of others reminds me of our common humanity.

I now know that I am not unique in my suffering. And just as the suffering I experience is not unique to me, the wisdom I have to share with others through my services is not unique to me either. What is unique to me is how I express the universal truths accessible by all. For instance, no one else can write this story as I do.

I used to make myself feel special by setting myself apart from everyone, but now I know that I am actually special because I am part of a very special whole.

The Highest Good of All

I've heard that life happens *for* me not *to* me. I agree that everything in this life, including our pains and our triggers, can be seen as opportunities to learn and evolve. But I prefer to say that life happens for us as a whole, as opposed to happening just for me, because it appears to me that this mysterious universe has not got just my back: it has our back.

Whether this belief is right or wrong, what matters to me is that meaning can be found in the possibility that the universe unfolds not just for me but for the highest good of our whole.

I was introduced to this concept of the highest good of all after learning that there is one common intention that healers set whether doing reiki or medical qigong. Before engaging in healing the healee, the healer must set the intention for the healing session to unfold not just for the highest healing possible to the healee that day, but also for the healing to be in line with the highest good of all.

Since the summer of 2017, I have been setting these intentions. Before I even get out of bed, I ask the divine for the following: 1) guidance for that day so that I may be a vessel of love, 2) protection of my physical, energetic, and spiritual bodies, 3) guidance so that my actions unfold toward the highest healing available to everyone and everything I come in relationship with that day, and 4) healing in line with the highest good of all.

I not only find this a simple practice of remembering our wholeness, but it also helps me to accept when things don't go as I plan. With a chronic condition of beating myself up when my daily goals are not met, remembering that my will may not always be in line with the highest good of all helps me to let go of my expectations when they're not met. While things may not seem to be going for my personal best, I try to trust that perhaps things are unfolding for the universal best.

I've met numerous people who have been able to turn their personal pains into universal gains. While I cannot share all of these stories, I will share that of Justina Marianayagam who, like me, has used her chronic pain as a platform to grow and be of service to a greater good.

Justina is a twenty-one-year-old who was diagnosed with widespread chronic pain syndrome when she was sixteen. I had the opportunity to connect with Justina at the Canadian Pain Society's 2017 Annual Scientific Meeting in Halifax, Nova Scotia. Justina's pains transformed her from a normal teenager whose only worry is to finish high school into a teenager who adopted the 3P approach (pharmacology, psychology, and physiotherapy) to manage her syndrome. Justina worked daily on her recovery, and over time she was able to go from being bedridden to a wheelchair, to using a walking stick, to walking on her own without gait aids.

Throughout the first stages of living with chronic pain, Justina relied heavily on pharmaceuticals, as she viewed illness through a biomedical lens and believed it was the only way to manage it. But as she explored others ways of coping, her lens on illness and wellness has broadened to encompass an appreciation for indigenous medicine and its integration. She was introduced to mindfulness by her psychologist at Sick Kids Hospital and started incorporating daily meditation with music and deep-breathing exercises to manage her pain. During severe pain flare-ups, she exchanged a bottle of painkillers for relaxation. Justina started to manage her pain with her mind— she did not want to have to rely on pharmaceuticals for the rest of her life, as they were disrupting her cognition and daily activities. It was a hard decision to make; it took autonomy as a pediatric patient being treated in a dominantly biomedical system. Following her diagnosis, her passion for healthcare spurred her and motivated her to graduate high school and enter university (despite those saying she would not be able to do so).

Justina is currently completing her BHSc as a 2014 Loran Scholar within the Faculty of Health Sciences at the University of Ottawa. Originally from Yellowknife, Justina moves forward with a strong passion for Northern health issues and health promotion through education. During the summer of 2017, she worked as a health policy analyst with the Institute for Circumpolar Health Research. She is working on a project that seeks to ensure indigenous patients have access to traditional medicinal care in a culturally respectful environment, without barriers, in all medical centres in the Northwest Territories. She is working alongside indigenous elders to promote the benefits of traditional medicine and ceremonies in improving the health of indigenous patients. Justina aspires to become a physician in the North and to promote two-eyed seeing and collaboration of traditional healing practices of indigenous people with Western practices.

I find great meaning in Justina's story, in that chronic pain did not happen *to* her—it happened *for* us and the highest good of our whole.

Make a Connection and Get Back to One

One day I met up with my friend Veronica at the Evergreen Brick Works Farmers Market. After purchasing some food we found a picnic table to sit down at, eat, and chat. A few minutes into our conversation, two women approached our table and sat at the other end. Veronica glanced over at an

African woven grocery basket that belonged to the woman beside her. Veronica turned to the woman and commented on how beautiful the basket looked, filled with a colourful array of fresh vegetables. What ensued was a conversation between the four of us that began with what the two women were going to have for dinner and transformed into a conversation about the practice of happiness, gratitude, and connection.

One of the women, whose name is Sharareh Vafai, went on to say what a beautiful soul her friend was. Knowing that not everyone I meet believes we have souls, I was intrigued to hear more about her experience of the soul, so I prompted her to share her perspectives on spirit. Sharareh shared her belief that at one point in time we were all together, and thus when we meet new people we actually don't have to do anything to get to know each other, because we already do know each other.

"We are all drops from the same source," Sharareh said. "The drop of the same spirit is in each of us. That's why we recognize ourselves in each other."

"Wow. So that's why one of my greatest experiences of joy is when a stranger looks directly into my eyes and shares a smile. It's because we are recognizing ourselves in the other!" I shared.

"We are all soul mates. We all carry that drop." Sharareh then went on to remind us that the term *namaste* does not just mean "the good in me sees the good in you"; it goes deeper, acknowledging spirit and how the divine drop in me sees the divine drop in you.

"Connect to the source and see that divine drop in yourself and in all our brothers and sisters, even those we are not fond of," Sharareh explained. "We are here to make a connection and get back to one."

Part V

An Overachiever Accepts What Can't Be Achieved

15

Healing as a Daily Practice

Wanting to Finish Healing

When I first embarked on this journey of healing I thought there was a finish line, a point where I'd be able to check off the tick box beside the task of healing on my to-do list and say, "I'm done! I did it! I have achieved healing!"

With a long ingrained habit of gaining my worthiness only through accomplishments and achievements, I could not accept the notion that there is no end point to healing. Underlying my attachment to finishing healing was a judgment toward my wounds as something that made me weak, beaten, and less than others. These intentions changed, however, as I came to learn that wounds are a natural part of living in this physical human form and perhaps the reasons why my soul chose me.

There's Always Going to Be Something

Up until my move to Vancouver five years after my accident, I was seeing my social worker Tracy Martin regularly six times a year. When the time came for my move, I called Tracy to ask for her opinion on whether we should go about continuing our sessions over the phone while I was away or if we should just move on to an as-needed basis. I told Tracy that I was afraid to end our sessions because it would somehow mean that I was done with the work of inner healing. Tracy let out a kind laugh and said that I would never be done.

"Never?" I asked in disbelief.

She then explained to me that as long as I keep creating the space for healing to happen, things will come up.

"There's always going to be something," she said.

So while I continue to find myself integrating parts of myself every day, healing is becoming a daily practice that I've accepted will be a lifelong practice.

It's a Spiralling Journey

I used to think that healing was a linear journey with clear start and end points. But after experiencing the various stages of healing personally, I have come to understand the healing journey as a spiralling one that moves both inwards and outwards: inwards within this human body and outwards beyond the physical self.

Can You Get Me There in Three Months?

I received the chiropractic method called NSA consistently from 2015 to 2017, both in Toronto and Vancouver. One thing that I appreciate about NSA is that the patient is asked to do homework to support the NSA work done on the treatment table. The homework I learned to do was based on the book of Donald M. Epstein, DC, *The 12 Stages of Healing: A Network Approach to Wholeness*.[8] Its exercises involve specific physical movements, touch, mantras, focused attention, and breathing patterns, self-prescribed according to which of the twelve stages of healing I happen to find myself in at any moment.

According to Dr. Epstein, the twelve stages of healing could also be thought of as the twelve stages of consciousness, with the greatest amount of suffering in stage one, and the highest level of conscious awareness and sense of connection with our communal wholeness occurring in stage twelve.

I recall sitting in the office of Dr. Barriscale during our first one-on-one meeting and asking her, "How many months will it take for you to get me to stage twelve? Can you get me there in three months?"

Dr. Barriscale very compassionately explained to me that healing is not about getting to the last stage but about meeting ourselves as we are, no matter the stage we are in. This did not sit well with me, because I had a lot judgment around being in stage one, where I often experience self-judgment, anger, fear, worry, confusion, and loneliness. I wanted to reach and live in stage twelve so I could just feel good at all times. Dr. Barriscale helped me to understand that as we continue to heal and evolve, it is normal for us to return often to the earlier stages, and it does not mean that we are regressing. With more wisdom and compassion embodied as we go through the stages of consciousness, we can return to the lower stages where suffering exists so that we can heal deeper and deeper wounds yet to be met.

Dr. Barriscale helped me to open up to the idea that healing is not about getting to enlightenment and feeling good all the time. Instead, we can practise reaching enlightenment so we can continue to bring the light and love of consciousness down to the darkest parts of our human experiences.

Get Me to the Final Level

When one of my girlfriends, Sadaf Ghezelbash, left her

career as an early childhood educator to become a certified professional coach, I was curious to receive her services. I had never worked with a coach before. During our first few sessions, Sadaf explained her role as a Master Practitioner of the Energy Leadership Index. She explained how she would work with me to help me understand my energetic profile according to the Core Energy Leadership Index developed by Bruce D. Schneider, a psychologist, master coach, and founder of iPEC Coaching.

Similar to Dr. Epstein's twelve stages of healing, where there is less suffering as one reaches higher stages, Schneider's seven levels of energy go from the least amount of available energy in level one to the highest amount of available energy in level seven. The lower stages of energy are described as catabolic (or in other words, destructive), with judgment, fear, and victimization keeping one's available power low. On the other hand, the higher levels of energy are described as anabolic (or in other words, positive), with much more power available through awareness, bliss, passion, and creativity.[9]

With my attachment to finishing healing and accomplishing growth, I clearly expressed my goals to Sadaf: "Sadaf, I need your services so you can get me to the final level."

Like Dr. Barriscale, Sadaf compassionately helped me to see how I was judging my experiences of lower levels of energy. I did not accept myself in all the colours of my human experiences. Sadaf helped me to understand that while I can continue to tap into the highest levels of energy through awareness practice and conscious choice making, it is important that I accept myself no matter what levels of energy I may find myself experiencing.

Spiral versus Circle

Unlike a circle, where one is just coming back to the same exact place, a spiral comes full circle but to a place with more depth and expansion. As we expand our loving awareness, we move up to new stages or levels of energy and healing, and we reconnect with our sense of wholeness and the mysterious love within all things. With the integration of this divine light, we continue along the spiralling journey, back down to the lower stages of suffering. It may appear we are back at square one, lost in confusion and disconnected from our wholeness, but we are not back to where we were. Instead, we are actually going deeper into the wounds of our humanity, whether they be of this lifetime, a past lifetime, or the lifetimes of our ancestors. Like peeling the layers of an onion or the layers of tree bark, we can meet our wounds one moment at a time. With expanding mindfulness and compassion we can go deeper, bringing divine love to heal the darkest parts of ourselves and consequently each other.

Now, I used to think that the path of healing was all sunshine and rainbows. After all, healing is supposed to be about love. But there is always yin to balance yang, and as my teacher Wendy Lang explained to me, the more light we receive, the more shadows we will discover. So alas the healing journey is not always a bright one. At times the healing path will be dark, illuminated only by the loving light that we choose to bring to it.

What Is Medicine Anyway?

If healing is a reconnection to our sense of wholeness, then good medicine will help us to become more whole. My own healing journey has been a humbling one that has opened me to receiving forms of medicine that my Newtonian mindset previously judged. With the opening qualities of mindfulness, I have come to integrate the medicine of emotional and energetic work and shamanism with my use of traditional Western medicine. Now, this integration is not so much a matter of incorporating both Eastern and Western forms of medicine, but a decolonization and indigenization of my perceptions of what can be considered medicine. Whether I am learning about the shamanic practices of China's earliest healers or the shamanic practices of the indigenous peoples of the Philippines and Turtle Island, I am discovering that there is much medicine to be learned from our elders and our teachers of ancient healing practices.

As a healthcare professional it is humbling for me to learn that one does not need to have an academic education to provide good medicine. To me, it seems most important that a healer exhibit wisdom, compassion, skilled energy work, and a deep, trusting connection to the spiritual source of love.

The Breath—the Ultimate Connector

If there is one common thread weaving all forms of healing practice together, I would say it is the use of the breath.

The word "spirit" comes from the Latin word *spiritus*, which actually means "breath." In Greek, the word for spirit is *pneuma*, which also means "breath," and in Hebrew, *Yahweh* means "wind." What's beautiful about the air we breathe and the air that blows in the wind is that air is the ultimate connector of all of life. Plants, animals, and humans are all connected through the air we breathe. Perhaps this is why, despite there being so many ways to meditate, all meditations involve the breath.

I use the breath to reconnect. When I breathe I can reconnect to the physical body and the emotions and energy moving (or not moving) through me. When I breathe I can reconnect with my true authentic higher self, my soul. When I breathe I can reconnect with our wholeness and the mystery of our ever-evolving love.

My soul entered this physical world with an inhale, and it will leave this world with an exhale. Between birth into this life and death from this life, it is through the breath that I am able to experience this being human. But it is also through the breath that I am able to remember and reconnect with the truth of who I really am.

When I breathe with these intentions to heal and return to wholeness, then breathing becomes a healing practice that I can engage in at any time, every day, no matter what I am doing. Every breath becomes an opportunity to cultivate the mindful ways of trust, patience, non-judgment, acceptance, beginner's mind, and the ability to let go. Every breath becomes an opportunity to respond with compassion.

What I love most about using breathing as a healing practice is that it does not require an insurance plan. Because the breath is always there, it is not something we can lose or forget at home. The breath is absolutely free, and thus it is a healing resource that is universally accessible. As long as we are still living, we can trust that the breath will be there like a loyal friend, connecting us to whatever source we trust in. For however we perceive the source of love, it is always accessible in the present moment through the breath.

Recovering Beyond

The most thought-provoking question I have ever been asked

is this: "Jaisa, how far are you in your recovery? For instance, what percentage have you recovered so far?"

For the first several years after the accident I would often reply with "Fifty percent, fifty-five percent, sixty-percent," and so on, as I progressed physically and functionally.

But if someone were to ask me that same question today I'd say, "I've recovered beyond one hundred percent of who I was before the accident, because I can now feel and embody life through more of my physical, energetic, and spiritual self than I ever did throughout my teens and my twenties."

Though it's been almost eight years since sustaining the spinal cord injury, my body is still showing progress. In the last year, I've been able to wean myself off wearing ankle foot orthoses, and I now only use high-stability runners and orthotics for arch support when I'm walking outdoors. For short distances indoors, I am able to function with only slippers, though with some minimal pain. Overall, I am able to stand on my feet longer, walk farther, and engage in more functional activities (such as carrying groceries) with less pain intensity as each year goes by.

I can confidently say that I am now living well with pain.

Perhaps more important than my physical and functional gains is the greater sense of connection to my inner truth. With the reclaiming of more of my soul and the reconnection to our spiritual wholeness, my daily self-care—or shall I say, my daily soul care—has become a non-negotiable. For now I know that through interconnectedness my own soul care is actually universal care. So I am committed to getting enough rest, water, and nourishing food. I meditate and pray daily and alternate between yoga, Pilates, and medical qigong. I do cardio and take hot Epsom salt baths several times a week. I seek the help of those I trust for physical, emotional, energetic, and shamanic work. And of course, I get outside to breathe fresh air every day.

There are still many goals that I am working toward, and they include learning to walk, jump, run, and dance barefoot again. But I am not attached to these goals, because I have come to peace with where I am today. Though it took a spinal cord injury for me to get out of my head and return to my body, I no longer suffer with chronic unworthiness. Now I live with a growing mindfulness and compassion for myself that allows me to accept and integrate all parts of who I am.

I am now more whole than who I was when the accident broke me.

I may not be able to walk barefoot just yet, but I do now know how to stand in the truth of who I am.

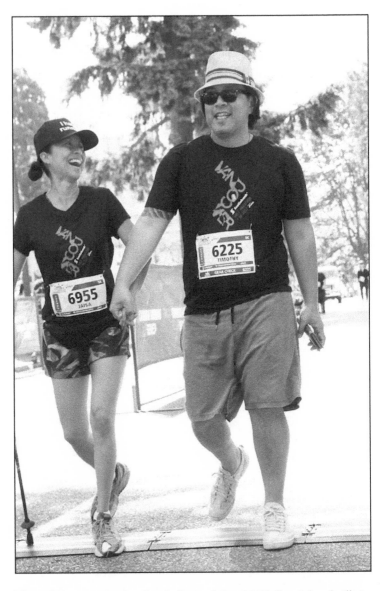

TJ and I crossing the finish line of the 2017 Scotiabank 5k in Vancouver in support of Spinal Cord Injury BC. I was able to complete the walk with one hiking stick, orthotic arch supports, and an authentic smile.

Acknowledgements

This book has unfolded as it has because of the guiding force of divine love that shows up in my life in many ways, including through the many people whom I'd like to thank.

First, I acknowledge my mother Luisa Baello Sulit and my father Jaime Chiu Sulit, whose unconditional love is the reason I know how powerful meaningful living can be. No one has given to me more than my parents have, and for that I am grateful.

To my ancestors, especially my Lola Lourdes Santos Baello and Lola Lily Chiu Sulit (*lola* means "grandmother" in Tagalog), thank you for watching over me. To the rest of my family, in particular the Baello, Lorenzana, and Santos families for showing me the medicine of a village. Special shout-out to my cousin Don Santos for telling me "You should write a book!"

To all my friends who believed in my ability to write, including Lynn Castro, who has gifted me with many journals, including the one I wrote in after the accident. To Catherine Caragan, Mayleen, Sean, and Charmaine Hew Wing for being my personal cheerleaders throughout the entire writing and publishing process. To Veronica Takes for the café dates where we would work on our books together. To June Son, whose pep talk one night led me to finalize my contract with my partner publisher the next day. To Melanie Cunanan, who helped me to get over myself so I could finally give my story an ending. To Karen Anzai, for being my *kalyāna-mittatā* and sharing this journey of awakening with me.

Thanks to my dream rehabilitation team: personal injury lawyers Greg Neinstein and Sonia Leith; case manager Ellie Lapowich; social worker Tracy Martin; physiotherapists

Kyle Whaley, Suzie Iafolla, Nathan Wong, Carole Chebaro, and Darryl Tracy; occupational therapists Holly Mo and Anat Barat; physiatrist Milan Unarket; chiropractors Blessyl Buan, Allison Barriscale, Nam Nguyen, Avi Sussman, and Joyce Chen; massage therapist Liezel Anne Palon; BodyTalk practitioner Linda Eales; reconnective healing practitioner Shawna Coudin; dietician Aimee Hayes; reflexologist Yvonne Osondu; shiatsu therapist Taichi Iwano; therapeutic writing group facilitator Melissa Melnitzer; professional coach Sadaf Ghezelbash; expressive arts therapist Andrea Mapili; feldenkrais practitioner May Nasser; somatic experiencing practitioner Jane Courtney; and naturopath Jenny Jun. Special thanks to Tracy, Kyle, Blessyl, Allison, Joyce, Liezel, Sadaf, Andrea, and Jane for the feedback on my writing and allowing me to share what transpired during our sessions.

To Jen Maramba, Babette Santos, Lorelei Williams, Kathara Pilipino Indigenous Arts Collective Society, and Butterflies in Spirit: thanks for opening my mind to the medicines of our ancestors. Thanks as well to Sharon Brant, Corrine Enojo and Justina Marianayagam, for allowing me to share their stories in this book.

I'd like to acknowledge Jon Kabat-Zinn, whose mindfulness work has not only helped me heal but has created a pathway for me to help others heal as well. Thanks to all the clients who have trusted me to facilitate their remembering of mindfulness, and to the participants of the mindfulness groups I've run. Their courage and openness to face challenges head-on inspires me to keep learning and growing.

To Dr. Ted Robinson, who took me on as an MBSR co-facilitator and provided me with mentorship, demonstrating the art of inquiry with wisdom and compassion. To the monthly mindfulness-for-chronic-pain group at Bridgepoint

Active Healthcare, especially those who have continued to return since the first year we began MBSR. I am grateful to be seen as a peer and be a part of this healing circle.

Thanks to Shari Stein for her guidance and open heart, and to Dr. David Etlin for generously allowing me to use his MBSR manuals for my courses and for reminding me to discuss suffering in this book. Thanks to Dr. Lucinda Sykes for her encouragement and belief that my story would benefit many.

I'd like to acknowledge Neal Pearson, whose work on pain care has helped me, and in turn my patients, to better understand the neurophysiology of the pain experience. Neil helped me to complete the section on "Turning toward the Pain = Gain." Thanks to Kristin Neff, whose research on self-compassion has helped me to cultivate a self-care routine. Kristin provided me with feedback on my sections on self-compassion in chapter seven.

Thanks to Suzanne Scurlock-Duranna, whose Healing from the Core workshops first introduced me to the reality of life force energy. To Wendy Lang at the Empty Mountain Institute, who always creates a safe space for me and my classmates to explore healing, and whose compassionate ways of teaching have helped me to see the divine in all things. Thanks to Wendy for supporting the completion of this book; her work has played a role in my transformation. A shout-out (or shall I say, "qi-out out") to my medical qigong classmates, who continue to support each other and the powerful work we are doing.

To the Sisterhood of Spiritual OTs: Avdeep Bahra, Kristina Borho, and Lynne Newman; thanks for exploring with me the role of spirit in occupational performance. Thanks to Trisha Dempsey for her electional astrology services, which have helped me to align the publishing of this book with the highest good of all.

To my friends Janet Walmsley and Jenny Story, whose books inspired me to pursue publishing as they did. Janet has been a resource for publishing and marketing advice and is the one who encouraged me to take Julie Salisbury's InspireABook Workshop in 2015. One year later, Julie became my partner publisher, and since then Julie has been holding my hand through the entire writing and publishing process. Thanks to Julie, who saw the necessity in me of sharing my story with the world; she motivated me to "just keep writing" whenever I was faced with the blocks of perfectionism. Because of Julie, I have benefited from being a part of her Authors of Influence Publishing community, which is also supported by Marilyn R. Wilson, who regularly shares resources on writing, publishing, and marketing.

Thanks to Greg Salisbury for his assistance with the publishing process, including typesetting, photo editing, and completion of the book cover. Thanks as well to illustrator Erin Taniguchi for creating the feathered yin and yang symbol on the front cover, and to Judith Mazari for assisting with cover design.

I'd like to thank the women of the Penning Divas, especially Evelyn McKelvie, Christine Awram, Diane Lund, and DeeAnn Lensen. I had the opportunity to meet these women at Julie Salisbury's InspireABook Workshop, after which we met regularly to support each other with the writing process.

To my editor Nina Shoroplova, whose guidance has helped me to move from writing with two different voices to writing with my one true voice. Thanks to Nina, I have been able to understand and thus share with clarity what my story is really about. Thanks as well to Rebecca Coates for her proofreading services.

Finally, to my life partner TJ Lim, who has provided me

with stability and support through the ups and downs of both the writing and the healing processes. I am grateful for his patience and understanding, and for his ability to make me laugh every day.

Glossary of Abbreviations

BHSc: bachelor in health sciences
CST: craniosacral therapy
DC: doctor of chiropractic
DTCM: doctor of traditional Chinese medicine
FFC: Folklorico Filipino Canada
MD: doctor of medicine
MBSR: mindfulness-based stress reduction
ND: naturopathic doctor
NLP: neuro-linguistic programming
NSA   Network Spinal Analysis
NYZCCC: New York Zen Center for Contemplative Care
OT: occupational therapy, occupational therapist
PhD: doctor of philosophy
PHE: physical health and education
SER: Somato-Emotional Release
SRI: Somato Respiratory Integration
TCM: traditional Chinese medicine
TRI: Toronto Rehabilitation Institute
U of T: University of Toronto
UV: ultraviolet

Notes

[1]Kabat-Zinn, J., E. Wheeler, T. Light, A. Skillings, M.J. Scharf, T.G. Cropley, D. Hosmer, and J.D. Bernhard. (1998). "Influence of a mindfulness meditation-based stress reduction intervention on rates of skin clearing in patients with moderate to severe psoriasis undergoing phototherapy (UVB) and photochemotherapy (PUVA)." *Psychosomatic Medicine*, Sep-Oct; 60 (5), 625–32.

[2]Pearson, N. (2008). *Understand Pain, Live Well Again.* Penticton, BC: Life is Now Pain Care Inc.

[3]Garland, E.L., E.G. Manusov, B. Froeliger, A. Kelly, J.M. Williams, and M.O. Howard, (2014). "Mindfulness-oriented recovery enhancement for chronic pain and prescription opioid misuse: Results from an early-stage randomized controlled trial." *Journal of Consulting and Clinical Psychology*, 82(3), 448–459.

[4]Neff, K.D. (2004). "Self-compassion and psychological well-being." *Constructivism in the Human Sciences*, 9, 27–37.

Neff, K.D. (2010). "Review of the mindful path to self-compassion: Freeing yourself from destructive thoughts and emotions." *British Journal of Psychology*, 101, 179–181.

Neff, K.D. (2011). "Self-compassion, self-esteem, and well-being." *Social and Personality Compass*, 5, 1–12.

Neff, K.D. (2012). "The science of self-compassion." In C. Germer & R. Siegel (Eds.), *Compassion and Wisdom in Psychotherapy*, 79–92. New York: Guilford Press.

Neff, K.D., K. Kirkpatrick, and S.S. Rude, (2007). "Self-compassion and its link to adaptive psychological functioning." *Journal of Research in Personality*, 41, 139–154.

Neff, K.D. and P. McGehee, (2010). "Self-compassion and psychological resilience among adolescents and young adults." *Self and Identity*, 9, 225–240.
Yarnell, L.M., & K.D. Neff, (2013). "Self-compassion, interpersonal conflict resolutions, and well-being." Self and Identity, 2(2), 146–159.

[5]Neff, K.D. and C.K. Germer, (2013) "A Pilot Study and Randomized Controlled Trial of the Mindful Self-Compassion Program." *Journal of Clinical Psychology*, 69: 28–44.

Baer, R.A. (2012). "Mindfulness and self-compassion as predictors of psychological wellbeing in long-term meditators and matched nonmeditators." *The Journal of Positive Psychology Dedicated to furthering research and promoting good practice*, 7(3), 230–238.

[6]Oriah "Mountain Dreamer" House from her book, THE INVITATION © 1999. Published by HarperONE, San Francisco. All rights reserved. Presented with permission of the author. www.oriah.org.

[7]Roman, S. & Packer, D. (1993). *Opening to Channel: How to Connect With Your Guide*. Novato, CA: HJ Kramer Publishing.

[8]Epstein, D.M. (1994). *The 12 Stages of Healing: A Network Approach to Wholeness*. San Rafael, CA: Amber Allen Publishing and New World Library.

[9]Schneider, B.D. (2007). *Energy Leadership: Transforming Your Workplace and Your Life from the Core*. Hoboken, NJ: John Wiley & Sons, Inc.

Author Biography

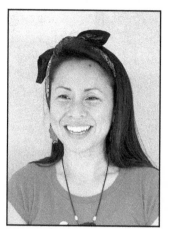

Jaisa Sulit is a registered occupational therapist who has been practising in Ontario since 2004. She is also a teacher who has held instructor and lecturer status at the University of Toronto's Department of Occupational Science and Occupational Therapy from 2005 to 2015.

While driving a motorcycle in 2010, Jaisa got into an accident that left her with a spinal cord injury and paralysis from the waist down. As a therapist-turned-patient, Jaisa integrated both traditional and non-traditional ways of healing. She completed a mindfulness-based stress reduction (MBSR) program that helped her to cope with stress, anxiety, depression, and chronic pain. Learning more than how to walk again, she learned how to reinhabit her body in ways she had never done before. Jaisa has gone on to become a qualified MBSR teacher through the Center for Mindfulness at the University of Massachusetts Medical School and has been teaching mindfulness to students, patients, and clinicians across Canada since 2012.

From 2015 to 2017, Jaisa lived in Vancouver, British Columbia, where she experienced the holistic benefits of daily connection with nature. Her curiosity led her to have a deeper understanding of her emotional-energetic body and how energy work and creative expression contribute to overall wellness. Jaisa has since completed certifications in reiki, medical qigong, and Chinese shamanic medicine and has become a keynote speaker, published poet and author.

Jaisa now lives in Toronto where she works as a holistic occupational therapist, integrating both science and spirit into her work. To connect with Jaisa and learn about her ongoing healing journey please visit www.jaisasulit.com and follow her on Instagram and Twitter @memoirsofajaisa.com.

About Jaisa

Jaisa offers a range of services and resources to help with your personal growth and healing journey:

- The Mindfulness-Based Stress Reduction course
- One on one mindfulness coaching in person, online or over the phone
- Retreats and workshops on mindfulness, compassion and medical qigong
- Medical qigong energy healing treatments in person or via distance sessions
- Keynote talks on mindfulness, wellness, healing and spirituality
- Free meditations uploaded weekly on her channel The Mindful Soul on the mindfulness app called Aura
- Free meditations on soundcloud.com/jaisa-sulit

To work with Jaisa or inquire about a possible speaking engagement please visit www.jaisasulit.com.

CPSIA information can be obtained
at www.ICGtesting.com
Printed in the USA
FSHW02n1956190618
49616FS

9 780995 984202